Springer
Tokyo
Berlin
Heidelberg
New York
Barcelona
Hong Kong
London
Milan
Paris
Singapore

Osamu Sugimoto

A Color Atlas of Hysteroscopy

With 277 Figures in Color

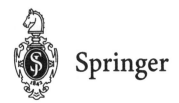

Springer

OSAMU SUGIMOTO, M.D., Ph.D.
Vice Director
Professor Emeritus of Osaka Medical College
19, Tsutsumicho, Nishikyogoku,
Ukyo-ku, Kyoto 615-0863, Japan

ISBN-13: 978-4-431-68393-3   e-ISBN-13: 978-4-431-68391-9
DOI: 10.1007/978-4-431-68391-9

Library of Congress Cataloging-in-Publication Data
Sugimoto, Osamu.
    A color atlas of hysteroscopy / Osamu Sugimoto.
        p.   cm.
    Rev. ed. of: Diagnostic and therapeutic hysteroscopy. 1st ed.
c1978.
    Includes bibliographical references and index.
    Rev. ed. of: Diagnostic and therapeutic hysteroscopy. 1st ed.
c1978.
    Includes bibliographical references and index.

paper)
    1. Hysteroscopy—Atlases.   2. Uterus—Diseases—Atlases.
I. Sugimoto, Osamu   Diagnostic and therapeutic hysteroscopy.
II. Title.
    [DNLM: 1. Uterine Diseases—diagnosis atlases.   2. Hysteroscopy—
methods atlases.   3. Cervix Diseases—diagnosis atlases.   WP17
S947c   1999]
RG304.5.H97S84   1999
618.1′407545—dc21
DNLM/DLC
for Library of Congress   98-37346

Printed on acid-free paper

© Springer-Verlag Tokyo 1999
Softcover reprint of the hardcover 1st edition 1999

SPIN: 10693300

Preface

In the first edition of *Diagnostic and Therapeutic Hysteroscopy* published in 1978 by Igaku-Shoin Ltd., the principal consideration was to demonstrate the superiority of diagnostic hysteroscopy by illustrating intrauterine abnormalities. Consequently, the emphasis was centered on instrumentation, diagnostic procedures, and the presentation of color photographs taken using still photography through a rigid water hysteroscope. Since that time, hysteroscopy has advanced remarkably thanks to a rapid expansion of indications for endoscopic surgery and to the progress in new instrumentation, including a flexible and steerable thin caliber fiber hysteroscope and the introduction of a new documentation system using TV monitoring.

At the same time, however, it has remained difficult to get a distinct picture of hysteroscopic findings on record because of the difficulties inherent in the use of a video camera with a fiber endoscope. While we have generally used TV monitoring for diagnostic hysteroscopy in accordance with current practice, we still insist on practicing still photography with a rigid hysteroscope to record precise images. We have always maintained that it is important to become proficient in using hysteroscopy as a diagnostic method before undertaking operative procedures. During the last few years, operative hysteroscopy has developed rapidly, and there are many relevant, up-to-date textbooks in this field. Consequently, operative hysteroscopy was not included in this atlas.

Since the publication of the first edition of this book, we have carried out 400 to 550 hysteroscopic examinations a year in patients with intrauterine abnormalities. In the course of these examinations, we have preserved quintessential diagnostic photographs of the diseases encountered. Almost all these hysteroscopic photographs, more than 200 of which appear in this book, were taken with an improved single-lens reflex camera (Olympus OM 2) connected directly to the eyepiece of a rigid hysteroscope. All pictures are remarkably clear, making any concomitant pen and ink illustrations unnecessary.

Osamu Sugimoto, M.D., Ph.D.

Contents

Fundamentals of Hysteroscopy

Hysteroscopic Findings of the Normal and Abnormal Uterus

Fundamentals of Hysteroscopy

1 Aim and Significance of Hysteroscopy

The uterus is an organ with highly hemorrhagic tendencies. Abnormal uterine bleeding is one of the most common gynecological disorders; it may result from various intrauterine abnormalities, and occurs regardless of the patient's age. The traditional gynecological examinations, including analysis of anamnesis, speculum and pelvic examination, cytology smears, and biopsies, do not always lead to correct diagnosis. Additional imaging techniques such as hysterography, ultrasonography, computed tomography (CT), and magnetic resonance imaging (MRI) may be equally equivocal.

The uterus is located in a short distance from the body surface and opens downward. The attempt to visualize lesions in the uterine cavity, namely, hysteroscopy, dates back more than 100 years when Pantaleoni reported the first successful hysteroscopy in 1869. He examined an endometrial polyp in a patient with postmenopausal uterine bleeding, inserting a simple hollow tube into the uterine cavity and illuminating the cavity with the candlelight reflected from a concave mirror. Other noteworthy events in endoscopy advances are the use of an optical lens system for the cystoscope originated by Nitze (1879) and an incandescent lamp at the tip of a cystoscope invented by Edison (1879). David (1908) was the first to apply Nitze's principle of an endoscope with a magnifying lens for hysteroscopy images.

With introduction of a lens system into hysteroscopic imaging, the contact type of hysteroscope has gradually turned into the panoramic mode. Unlike other hollow organs, the uterus is rather an unsuitable organ for endoscopic examination. Proper distension of the uterine cavity using positive-pressure medium is essential for clear panoramic visualization because the uterus is a hollow organ consisting of a thick and rigid muscle. Furthermore, the uterine cavity is lined with an endometrium that varies in thickness during the menstrual cycle and bleeds easily on contact.

Two general types of media, gas and liquid, have been used for uterine distension. Rubin (1925), who noticed uterine distension at the time of tubal insufflation under CO_2 pressure, made practical use of the gas as a distending medium during hysteroscopy for the first time. However, because several cases resulted in pneumoperitoneum, the method was abandoned until resurrected by Lindemann in Germany (1974) and Porto in France (1970). Since Seymour (1926), and Mikulicz-Radecki and Freund (1927) used liquid not only to flush blood and mucus from the uterine cavity but also to distend the uterus, the liquid-type hysterocope has been reported by many investigators, such as Gaus (1928), Schroeder (1934), Norment (1951), Englund et al. (1957), and many Japanese research workers. Schroeder reported interesting data on the intrauterine pressure suitable for liquid hysteroscopy; he found that the uterus required gravity pressures of 650 mm above the patient's intrauterine pressure for its distension, while a pressure higher than 950 mm of water led to peritoneal spillage through the tube.

Dextran 70 (Hyskon, Pharmacia), a highly viscous dextran solution, was adopted by Edstroem and Fernstroem (1970); this distending solution has several advantages, such as mixing only slightly with blood, thereby retaining its transparency throughout hysteroscopy, and it also reduces peritoneal leakage.

Norment (1943) reported a new technique wherein illumination is provided from an external light source through a glass fiber-optic bundle. This epoch-making attempt by Norment has enabled us to illuminate the intrauterine target with much more powerful cool light from a illumination source than that provided by the traditional distal electric incandescent bulb. Since that time, this system of illumination has been become standard for the hysteroscope. Moreover, advent of the 35-mm single lens reflex camera and "daylight" fast color film has made image recording simple and easy.

The current use of the video camera has brought an evolution in endoscopic documentation. Magnetic and optical devices and instant thermal printers can be coupled to a monitor; it is possible to reproduce and analyze the data obtained immediately after an examination.

Nowadays, fiber-optic bundles are used not only as a light guide but also for image transmission; a hysterofiberscope can be used to observe the lateral portion of the uterus because of its steerability and the flexibility of the distal end. The thin hysterofiberscope has a 4-mm OD (outer diameter) and is widely used during office diagnostic procedures in Japan. However, the image of the optic fiber hysteroscope is inferior to images from the rigid endoscope in sharpness.

Although operative hysteroscopy has recently received increased acceptance, the skills required and mastery of the techniques involved in learning diagnostic hysteroscopy to know intimately every view in the intrauterine milieu, normal and abnormal, must always precede operative hysteroscopic procedure.

Because the aim of *A Color Atlas of Hysteroscopy* is to print panoramic pictures as sharply and clearly as possible, all the photographs in this volume were taken by a 35-mm single reflex still camera using the rigid hysteroscope under liquid irrigation.

2 The Panoramic Hysteroscope

As already described, the uterus is essentially an unsuitable organ for endoscopic procedures: without mechanical dilatation, the isthmus is too narrow to introduce the endoscope; the uterine cavity is virtual, i.e., the two thick and rigid walls are in proximity with a narrow space; also, the endometrium is extremely fragile and easily hemorrhages on slight contact. To attain a distinct panoramic visualization using hysteroscopy, satisfactory uterine distension by positive pressure of a transparent medium and elimination of the blood, mucus, and debris that obstruct the view are required. The principles of panoramic hysteroscopy depend on interpretation of the location, extension, shape, contours, relief, colors, vasculature, consistency, and mobility of the lesions within the uterus. Most commonly used modern panoramic hysteroscopes can be divided into two major types: the rigid type and flexible type of instrument, according to the method of image transmission. Each has advantages and disadvantages, as shown in Table 1. The basic equipment of diagnostic hysteroscopy consists of four items: the hysteroscope, a light source, a light-transmitting glass fiber cable, and a suitable recording device (still cameras and video cameras).

Table 1. Strong and weak points of rigid and flexible hysteroscopes

	Rigid	Flexible
Image guide	Rod lens	Optic fiber bundle
Light guide	Fiber bundle	Fiber bundle
direction of vision	Direct or oblique	Steerable
Clarity of image	Sharp and clear	Dotted, distinct
Operation of tool	Easy	Rather complicated
Focus	Fixed	Adjustable
Price of tool	Moderate	Expensive

2.1 The Rigid Hysteroscope

The hysteroscope consists of a telescope and an outer sleeve with an obturator. The Olympus hysteroscope, our favorite (Fig. 1a,b), has an oval cross section of 4.0 × 6.3 mm, equipped with a Hopkins lens system with direct vision over a 60° visual angle and a fixed focal length of 2 mm. A light-transmitting cable, connecting the light source and the hysteroscope, consists of about 9000 optical glass fibers. The distal ends of the glass fibers are confined within the hysteroscope, surrounding the optic lens channel. There is one more thin channel, 2 mm in diameter, for water rinsing to dilate the uterine cavity, connecting to the inlet valve. The valve at the neck of the telescope regulates water intake from the irrigator at a height of 50 cm. The outer sleeve, a thin-walled cylindrical pipe, is 7 mm OD, and 2 mm longer than the telescope. It plays an important role in protecting the endometrium from direct contact with the telescope as well as keeping the distal lens at a fixed distance from the objects. A gap between the telescope and the outer sleeve is used as a channel through which sterile saline or 32% dextran solution is drained after lavage and distension of the uterine cavity.

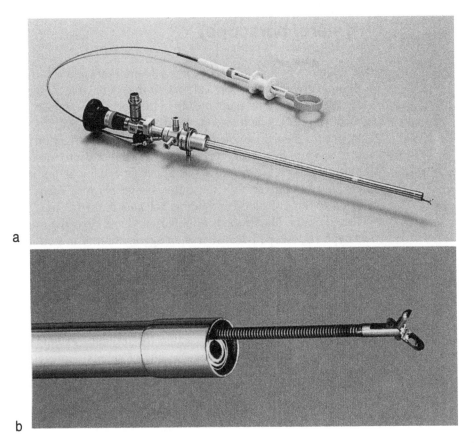

a

b

Fig. 1a,b. Diagnostic rigid hysteroscope (Olympus). **a** The endoscope is fitted into the outer sleeve. A flexible biopsy forceps is inserted in an irrigating channel. **b** Close-up view of the tip of the hysteroscope. The outer sleeve is 2mm longer than the endoscope. The biopsy forceps appear from the irrigating channel

2.2 The Steerable Hysteroscope (Hysterofiberscope)

The Olympus hysterofiberscope has a 3.5-mm OD and is 540 mm in length. It is equipped with a fiber-optical system that is flexible at the distal end and steerable through a total arc of 200° in the horizontal plane by using a manual control (Fig. 2a). The telescope has three channels, one for image transmission, one for the light guide, and the third for water irrigation (Fig. 2b). As the tool is thin and flexible, it is possible to see directly into the entire interior of the uterus. However, because the hysterofiberscope is not equipped with a drainage channel through the outer sleeve because of its flexibility, it is difficult to remove blood and debris masking the structures. Also, the image reflected on the fiberscope is less sharp and less clear than that on the rigid-lens-type endoscope because it is an aggregation of dotted images reflected through individual fibers (Fig. 3a,b). The Strong and weak points of each hysteroscope are described in Table 1.

There are a few other hysteroscopes, including the microcolpo-hysteroscope (Hamou; Fig. 4), needle hysteroscope, and operating hysteroscope, which are designed according to each clinical application. We have used either a fiberhysteroscope for ordinary examination or a rigid hysteroscope for photographic recording of valuable images of rare disease conditions.

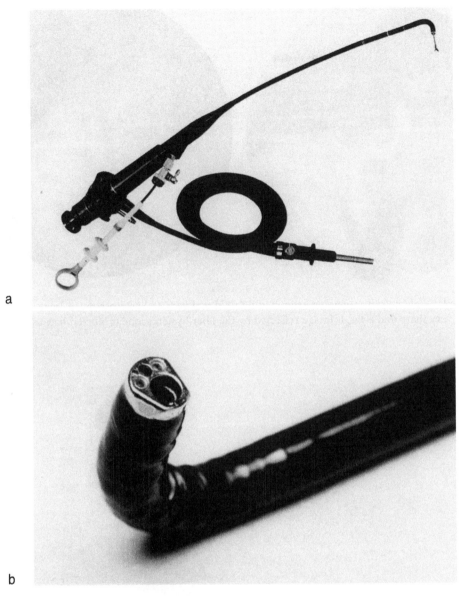

a

b

Fig. 2a,b. Steerable hysterofiberscope (Olympus). **a** This instrument is steerable and flexible at 2 cm of the distal end of the fiberscope (right and left) by hand control. **b** Close-up view of the tip of the fiberhysteroscope. The tip of the distal end, bent at a right angle, has two channels, an objective lens and a water-instilling one

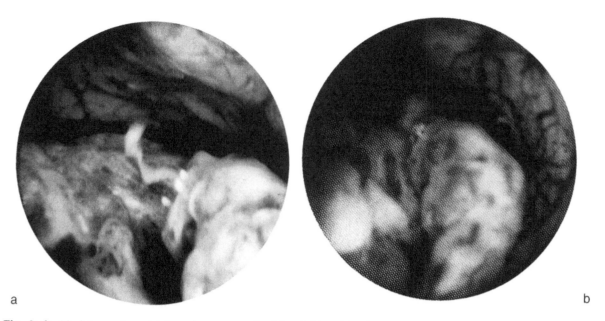

Fig. 3a,b. Nodular endometrial carcinoma examined by rigid and flexible hysteroscopy. **a** Image taken by the rigid hysteroscope is very sharp and clear. **b** Image reflected by the fiber hysteroscope is blurred because of low resolution

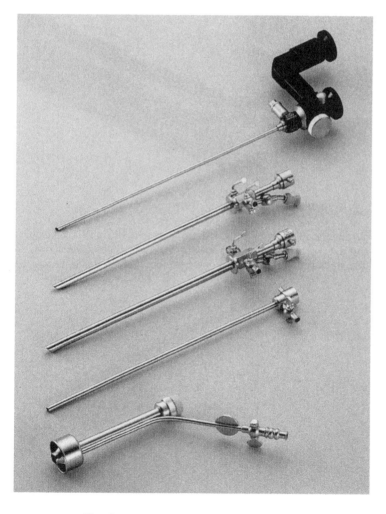

Fig. 4. Hamou's microcolpohysteroscope

3 Distension Media

To obtain a clear panoramic view of the uterine cavity, it is necessary to dilate the uterine cavity suitably with transparent media. Two kinds of media are now available for distension of the uterus, either liquid or gas. One liquid media is a physiologically isotonic solusion such as saline and 5% dextrose in water, and another is a highly viscous solution such as 32% dextran in dextrose (Hyskon). On the other hand, CO_2 has been used for gas hysteroscopy in Europe and America. The merits and demerits of each medium are described in Table 2. We personally prefer liquid hysteroscopy, particularly by dextrose solution or saline, for the following reasons: (1) a saline or dextrose solution is more efficient than gas for removal of blood, mucus, and debris that obstruct the view; (2) the detailed view of the lining of the uterine cavity when dilated by CO_2 insulation is obscured by the glare of the reflected light and by blood and mucus covering the surface of the lesions; (3) leakage of fluid through the fallopian tubes into the abdominal cavity is less than that of CO_2 because of its higher viscosity; and (4) because isotonic fluid media are used, soft structures such as an endometrial polyp and endometrial carcinoma appear vividly, swaying in the media, while CO_2 insufflation makes these tissues stick to the uterine wall, giving an unreliable view. On the other hand, a gas makes it easier to see the lesions in the right perspective. Figures 5a,b to 7a,b show pictures of an endometrial polyp, submucosal leiomyoma, and endometrial carcinoma in the same location of each lesion when comparing saline and CO_2 hysteroscopy, respectively.

Table 2. Characteristics of distension media in hysteroscopy

	Liquid		Gas
Media used	Physiological saline 5% glucose solution 3% D sorbitol solution 5% dextran solution	Hyskon	CO_2
Elimination of blood and debris in uterus	Easy	Difficult	Difficult
Vivid view of lesions	Easily obtained		Often obscured by glare
Perspective	Less correct	Correct	Correct
Leakage of media through tubes	Less	Least	Much
Embolism of media	None	None	Possible

We usually use saline or 5% dextrose solution and occasionally a highly viscous dextran solution. Most of the hysteroscopic pictures in this book were obtained under uterine distension by isotonic fluid media. The practical procedure of uterine distension is described in Fig. 8. Saline or 5% dextrose solution is delivered by simple gravity flow from the irrigator, which is raised 50–70 cm above the patient to obtain suitable pressure to distend as well as to irrigate the uterine cavity. When the distension is insufficient, additional solution may be instilled by using a 50-ml syringe through the three-way valve attached to the irrigation tube. The intrauterine pressure is adjusted by opening and closing the outflow valve while observing visual control.

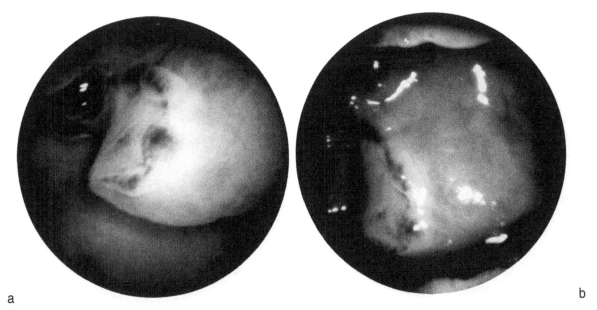

a

b

Fig. 5a,b. Endometrial polyp examined by water and CO_2 hysteroscopy. Age 43 years. C.C. (chief complaint): Menometrorrhagia. **a** The uterus is distended by saline. An endometrial polyp shows a conelike projection from the left cornu of which the surface is smooth and has no vascular pattern. On the *left side* an air bubble can be seen. **b** Endometrial polyp examined by CO_2 hysteroscopy. The uterus is dilated by CO_2 gas. The surface of the polyp has a glare from the lighting, resulting in an unclear view

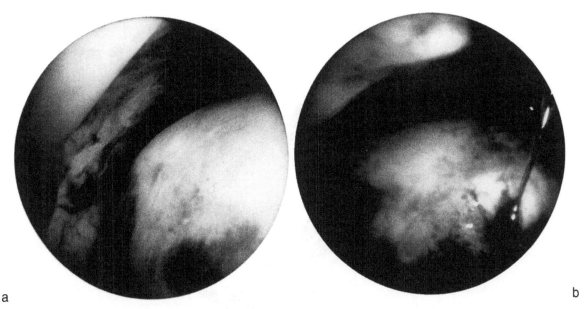

a

b

Fig. 6a,b. Submucosal fibroid examined by water and CO_2 hysteroscopy. Age 38. C.C.: Menometrorrhagia. **a** The uterus is distended by saline. After intrauterine blood clots have been washed out, the hysteroscopic view shows a spheric nodule of submucosal leiomyoma with smooth and ischemic surface. On part of the surface a tiny blood spot can be seen. **b** The uterus is distended by CO_2 gas. A hard tumor such as a fibroid shows a fairly clear view even by gas hysteroscopy, if blood coating on the surface is not dense

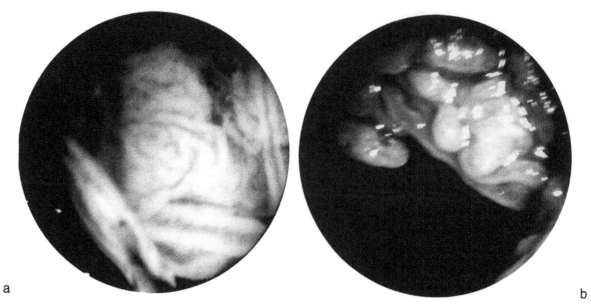

a   b

Fig. 7a,b. Papillomatous endometrial carcinoma examined by water and CO_2 hysteroscopy. Age 60. C.C.: Postmenopausal bleeding. **a** The uterus is dilated by saline. Some tentacles like projections with central vessels can be seen hanging down and swaying in the fluid medium. **b** CO_2 gas is used as the distending medium. Because the cancer tissue is not only collapsed and sticking to itself but also is covered with blood and mucus, the hysteroscopic view provides insufficient characteristics to mark endometrial carcinoma

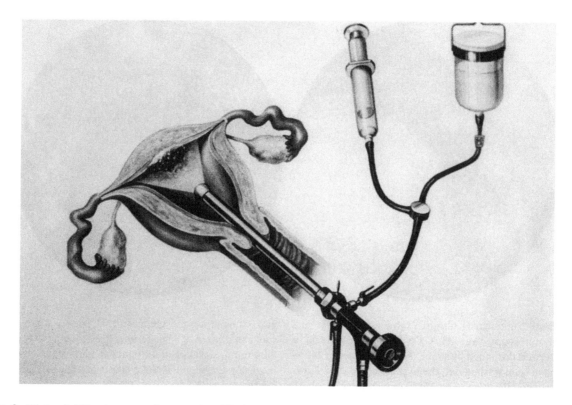

Fig. 8. Water rigid hysteroscopy in operation. The hysteroscope connected with a water irrigation apparatus is inserted in the uterine cavity. The irrigator, filled with rinsing fluid, is hung 50 cm above the patient

4 Practice of Panoramic Hysteroscopy

Modern panoramic hysteroscopy has now overcome many difficulties and has entered upon a new stage of practical use. The practical procedures done with a view to simple, safe, and efficient examination in the office are as follows.

4.1 Time of Practice

Hysteroscopy for the patient of reproductive age may be ordinarily best performed at some time after menstruation when the uterine cavity is lined with thin endometrium, is free of blood and debris, and is liable to distend even when using low-pressure rinsing fluid. The patient with abnormal bleeding should be examined just during her episode of bleeding before cell and tissue sampling to obtain an accurate visualization of the lesions.

4.2 Instrument Preparation

A set of hysteroscope, 35-mm single lens reflex still camera, video camera, video recording equipment and documentation, light source, 2-l irrigator, speculum, tenaculum, 5% dextrose solution or saline, and 1% Xylocaine are required.

4.3 Hysteroscopy Procedures

The patient is placed in a dorsal recumbent position (lithotomy position). The vagina is opened with a speculum and is disinfected with an appropriate antiseptic solution. Local anesthesia is optional. When the patient is nulliparous or postmenopausal and the cervical canal is very narrow, 10–15 ml of 1% Xylocaine may be administered for paracervical block. Multiparous patients usually do not require anesthesia.

4.3.1 Examination of the Intracervical Canal and Uterine Cavity

The examination is begun in the cervical canal without mechanical dilatation of the cervix. The hysterocope is fitted into the outer sleeve, the still or video camera is installed, and the inflow and outflow tubes are connected to the light source in advance. The instrument is then introduced into the external cervical os while irrigation is flowing through the hysteroscope under visual control. As the hysteroscope is gradually advanced, the cervical canal is dilated and exposed in its totality. Then the hysteroscope in the outer sleeve is temporarily pulled out of the cervix, and is replaced with an obturator. After the instrument is reintroduced just beyond the level of the internal cervical os, the obturator is changed for the hysteroscope at this point.

When the cervix is too narrow and rigid to insert the instrument atraumatically, it must be gradually distended to 7 mm in diameter by using a tapered dilator in advance. Visualization of the uterine cavity is systematically performed from the lower portion to the fundus and bilateral cornua under the optimum condition of its moderate dilatation by the pressure of the rinsing fluid. During the examination, care should be taken not to cause serious injury to the surface of the lesion(s) resulting from undue manipulation, thereby causing an interrupted view from unexpected bleeding.

4.4 Special Manipulation Techniques for Optimal Visualization

4.4.1 Visualization of the Difficult-to-Dilate Uterine Cavity

The relative difficulty of uterine distension under 50cm H_2O of gravity pressure depends on individual variation. On one hand, it varies according to age, the time of the menstrual cycle, and the kind of uterine lesions present in a patient. On the other hand, it is fairly easy in postmenopausal women who have a thin uterine wall. For the patient presenting with a uterus that is difficult to distend, the same solution used for irrigation or a highly viscous dextran solution (Hyskon) may be slowly instilled by using a 50-ml syringe through the three-way valve connected to the main inflow irrigation tube. Instillation pressure is adjusted under visual control so as not to be raised too much.

4.4.2 Visualization at the Time of Persistent Bleeding

Abnormal uterine bleeding is one of the most common gynecological disorders and the most frequent indication for diagnostic hysteroscopy. It is very important to perform the hysteroscopy concomitantly with an episode of bleeding to ensure its diagnostic and therapeutic efficacy. The procedure(s) for hysteroscopic examination of the uterine cavity with copious bleeding present requires great skill, because profuse bleeding causes poor vision. At this time fluid irrigation is patiently continued by fully opening the outflow valve to clear the uterine cavity of blood and debris. Most of the patients with bleeding can be satisfactorily examined by this procedure. When isotonic liquid media fail, however, Hyskon may be substituted for these media, being instilled through the three-way valve. Hyskon, a 32% dextran solution with a crystal-clear appearance, mixes poorly with blood because of its high viscosity, and so suppresses slight venous bleeding adequately as to provide a clear field of view.

4.4.3 Visualization of a Large Tumor

Endometrial polyps and submucosal leiomyoma occasionally may occupy a large area in the uterine cavity. The ordinary panoramic hysteroscope cannot view such a large tumor in its entirety in one field of vision. A definite procedure must be followed to picture the mental correction of its totality. The tumor usually appears as a round protrusion bulging toward the uterine cavity. The observation begins at the lower pole of the tumor and is followed clockwise, while the hysteroscope is slowly advanced from the posterior surface toward the fundus, confirming whether the tumor is pedunculated or sessile, and if pedunculated, where is the location and what is the thickness of the pedicle.

4.5 Hysteroscopic Biopsy

After a thorough examination of the uterine cavity using hysteroscopy, biopsy sampling for histological evaluation should be performed in some of the intrauterine diseases such as endometrial hyperplasia and endometrial carcinoma. The most ideal method is to sample the tissue sufficiently for the pathologist to interpret under hysteroscopic guidance. However, because the biopsy is usually performed with a flexible or semirigid forceps, the volume of tissue obtained is too small for correct diagnosis. We prefer the following technique; first, hysteroscopy identifies the lesion to establish a presumptive diagnosis as well as to specify the localization of the disease; second, the hysteroscope is then withdrawn, a rather large curette is directed to the known site of the lesion, and a sufficient sample of tissue is removed. It is important to histologically evaluate the disease appearance near the surface. In particular, a beginner in hysteroscopy should learn that the hysteroscopic findings of a particular disease mirror the characteristic histological organization, gaining many kinds of experience to compare both findings of the same site of the lesion.

Thus, the scrutiny of panoramic hysteroscopy after much experience enables us to roughly infer the histological appearance near the surface of the intrauterine lesion from its macroscopic appearance during the hysteroscopy.

4.6 Hysteroscopy Documentation

The findings obtained from hysteroscopic examination are recorded on still photographs or a video system, while the patient's chart documenting simple diagrams of the findings has another significant advantage. This document contains the patient's history and previous results of such procedures as a blind biopsy, hysterogram, and sonogram. Other essentials are the type of anesthesia, the method of cervical dilatation, and the type of distending media. Abnormal findings are documented in detail on every segment of the uterus, divided adequately. Finally, the hysteroscopic diagnosis and the histological results are put to good use for the design of future treatment (Fig. 9).

The 35-mm single lens reflex camera has been widely used as a most reliable means for correct recording of the hysteroscopic examination. It allows for excellent and maximum fidelity images of high-sensitivity daylight color film (Kodak, Ektachrome, ASA 400) for still photography can be used with shorter shutter speeds under the brightest possible illumination. The film is sensitive not only at the lesion but also at the border between the lesion and the surrounding normal region from various angles. The lesion is recorded in detail by using the approach shot and panoramically by using the bird's-eye view. When the hysteroscopic pictures obtained are filed together with the picture of the excised specimen and its histopathology, it is advantageous for easy cross-referencing of relevant data.

Takeda General Hospital Dep. OB/GYN

Hysteroscopy Report

Name *O.S.* Age *35* Date *07/20/ '96*

Clinical Symptoms: *Menorrhagia*

LMP: *07/05/* ~ *10* Days   Date of Cycle   Day *16*

Past Pregnancy: Gravidity *3* , Parity *2*

Recent Bleeding

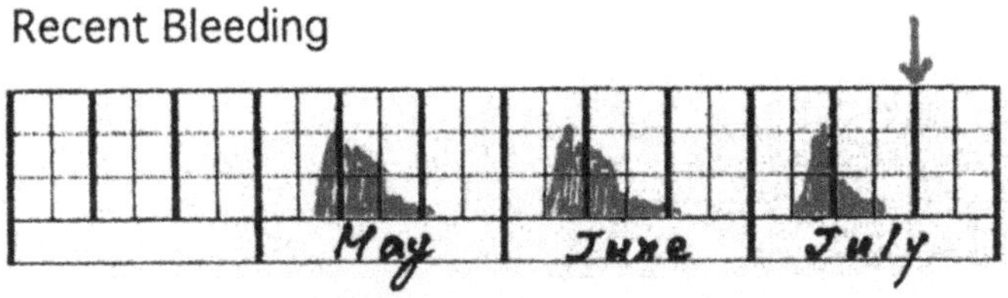

Previous Exam.

UCG	/	/
HSG	/	/
Biopsy	/	/
HCG	/	/

Findings: Ut.; antefl., retrofl., Cavity Length *7* cm

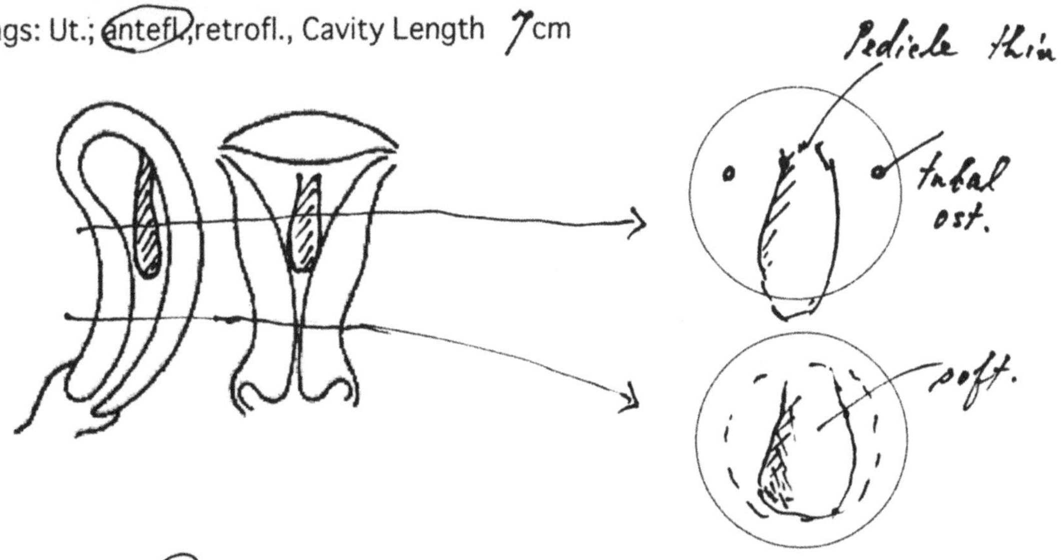

Anesthesia: Yes (No) (Type   )

Disted.Med.: (Saline), Dextrose or Hyskon

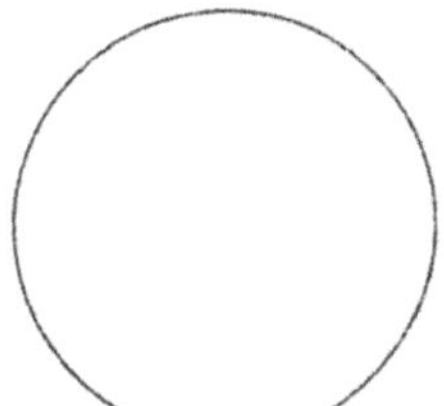

Cerv.Dilat.: Hegar No.   , Laminaria

Biopsy: (Yes) No   Hysteroscop. Diag. *Endometrial polyp*

Histolog. Diag.: *Endometrial polyp*

Further Treat. *Vag. polypectomy*

Signature *C. Sugimoto*

Fig. 9. Documentation chart used in our clinic (an example)

Video tape recording is useful for dynamic expression of the intrauterine spectacle, vividly presenting the location and extent of the lesion and its mutual relation to the surrounding structure. The advent of the still video recorder enables us to provide instant color prints. Such a vivid picture printed immediately after examination is useful in many ways, including the mutual communication between the physician and the patient. Recently a system unit, which is equipped with monitoring TV, light source, image processor, VTR, instant video printer, and hard copy system of still photography, has become available (Fig. 10a,b).

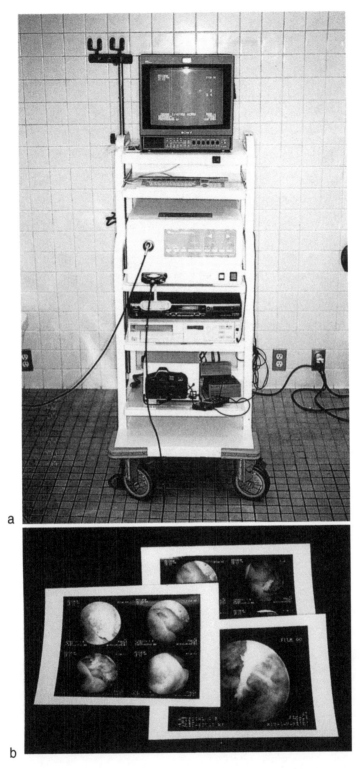

a

b

Fig. 10a,b. A set of light source and documentation apparatus of hysteroscope and instant color print. **a** By use of this apparatus, still photograph, video tape recording, and instant color print can be selected according to our preference. **b** Instant color print. Because pictures are printed immediately during examination, it is very useful for the patient in obtaining information about her disease from the physician

5 Indications and Contraindications

5.1 Clinical Indications for Hysteroscopy

Hysteroscopy has become the most accurate method available to evaluate intrauterine abnormalities. The development of instrumentation, technical refinements, and extensive clinical experience have increased the applicability of diagnostic, follow-up, and operative hysteroscopy. The present indications for hysteroscopy are as follows.

A. Diagnostic Hysteroscopy
   1. Symptomatological abnormalities
      i. Abnormal uterine bleeding (menorrhagia, metrorrhagia, peri- and postmenopausal bleeding, and contact bleeding)
         a. Intracervical abnormalities: endocervical polyps, cervical lacerations, cervical pregnancy, and intracervical carcinoma
         b. Intrauterine abnormalities: dysfunctional bleeding, retained secundines, trophoblastic diseases, tubal pregnancy, intrauterine foreign bodies, endometrial hyperplasia, endometrial malignancy, endometrial polyps, and submucosal myoma
      ii. Past intrauterine operations (miscarriage, legal abortion, cesarean section, insertion of an IUD (intrauterine device), myomectomy, and polypectomy)
         a. Intrauterine synechia
         b. Recurrence of submucosal leiomyoma and endometrial polyp
         c. Foreign bodies (IUD and threads)
   2. Intrauterine abnormalities suspected from traditional diagnostic methods
      i. Abnormal hysterogram
         a. Irregular contour: intrauterine adhesions, endometrial polyposis, endometrial tuberculosis, adenomyosis, endometrial hyperplasia, and endometrial carcinoma
         b. Filling defect: endometrial polyp, submucosal or pedunculated leiomyoma, intrauterine adhesions, and endometrial carcinoma
         c. Deformed contour: submucosal myoma
         d. Intravasation: chronic endometritis, endometrial tuberculosis, and adenomyosis
         e. Anomalous uterus
      ii. Miscellaneous
         a. Abnormal uterine biopsy (by blind curettage): chronic endometritis (foreign bodies, endometrial polyp, retained secundines, and endometrial carcinoma) and endometrial hyperplasia (endometrial polyps and submucosal leiomyoma)
         b. Abnormal uterine sounding: submucosal leiomyoma, intrauterine adhesions, and uterine malformation

        c. Abnormal image technology: submucosal leiomyoma, endo-
          metrial polyps, and endometrial carcinoma
    3. Infertility of unknown cause
  B. Follow-up hysteroscopy
    1. Follow-up after conservative surgery for intrauterine lesions:
       polypectomy, myomectomy, synechiotomy, and plastic surgery of
       malformed uterus
    2. Follow-up after medical treatment of endometrial hyperplasia
    3. Follow-up after irradiation for endometrial carcinoma
  C. Operative hysteroscopy
    1. Biopsy under visual control: endocervix, endometrium, and fetal
       elements
    2. Polypectomy, myomectomy, synechiotomy, and resection of uterine
       septum
    3. Endometrial ablation for persistent bleeding

5.2 Contraindications for Hysteroscopy

Contraindications for hysteroscopy have now decreased owing to the im-
provement of the instrumentation and the endoscopist's dexterity. However,
an examination performed on a patient with an active pelvic infection,
especially acute endometritis and cervicitis, should be contraindicated for
hysteroscopy until the inflammation subsides. Otherwise, the patient is in
danger of spreading infection and exacerbation of the condition. When
pyometra is suspected, however, hysteroscopy may be somewhat recommended because cervical dilatation promotes pus drainage.

Intrauterine pregnancy is a contraindication for hysteroscopy because of
the dangers of causing infection to the early fetus and interrupting a desired
pregnancy.

Profuse uterine bleeding is usually not a contraindication. The uterine
cavity is patiently irrigated with a suitable rinsing fluid until the returning
fluid is clear. Consequently, the slightly high pressure of the fluid in the
uterine cavity makes it possible to obtain a clear view.

Hysteroscopic Findings of the Normal and Abnormal Uterus

6 The Cervix

First of all, initial observation by hysteroscopy should be begun in the cervical canal before mechanical dilatation of the cervix. The cervical canal, which measures 2–3 cm from the external to the internal os in length, is lined by the endocervix with a *pink-white* color and a complicated wrinkle pattern. Once the instrument and hysteroscope are prepared for an efficient examination, the hysteroscope is advanced slowly from the external os into the cervical canal under visual control. The cervical canal results in the entire scene as the pressure of the rinsing fluid increases gradually by turning off the outflow valve. To get useful information about endocervical pathology by using hysteroscopy, it is necessary to know the normal findings of the cervical canal in advance.

6.1 Normal Findings of the Cervix

In nulliparous reproductive-age women, the inner surface of the cervical canal resembles numerous fern leaflike folds or a branched crest, the so-called plica palmatae (Figs. 11, 12). The pattern of the folds may appear individually either dense or thin (Figs. 13, 14). The relief of the folds is tinged with a *light pink* or *whitish-yellow* color and is *translucent.*

In multiparae, these are somewhat attenuated (Fig. 15), and in postmenopausal women they become more flattened, atrophic, and *pale* (Fig. 16).

The internal os, a constricted part between the cervical canal and uterine cavity, is a smooth and narrow circle under uterine distension by using irrigation (Figs. 17, 18).

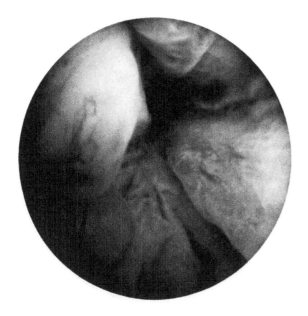

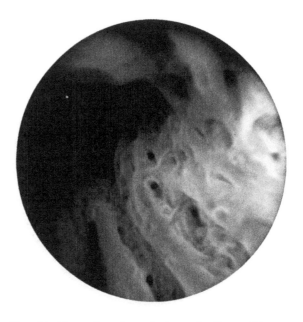

Fig. 11. Normal endocervical canal of a nulliparous woman. Age 25. Several longitudinal crests with uneven surface and shaggy subepithelial vessels converge on the internal os. The plicae palmatae are well preserved

Fig. 12. Normal endocervical canal of a nulliparous woman. Age 30. Some crests have crypts of various sizes

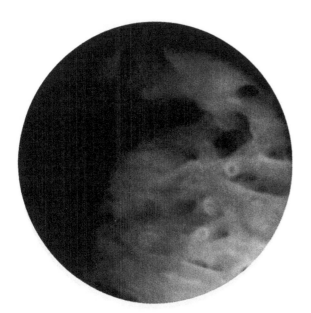

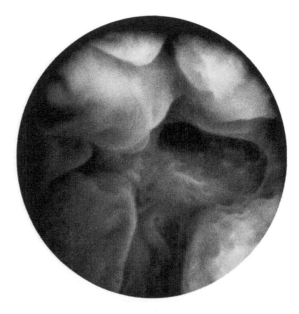

Fig. 13. Normal endocervical canal of a nulliparous woman. Age 26. The plicae are somewhat irregular and decreased

Fig. 14. Normal endocervical canal of a multiparous woman. Age 27. The crests form complicatedly branched trabeculae

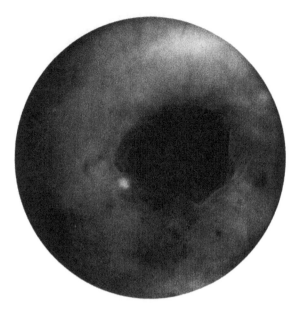

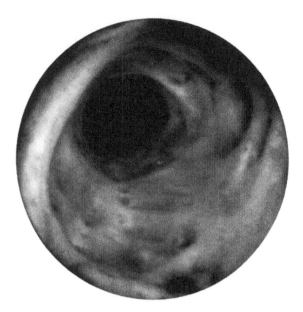

Fig. 15. Normal endocervical canal of a multiparous woman. Age 47. The cervical mucosa, of which the surface has a few glandular openings, show relief from the folds

Fig. 16. Normal endocervical canal of a postmenopausal woman. Age 55. The scarred cervix is lined with annular crests

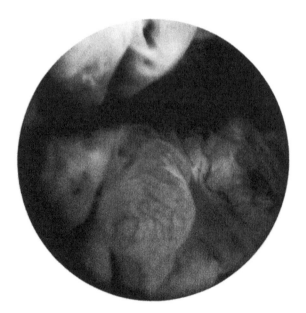

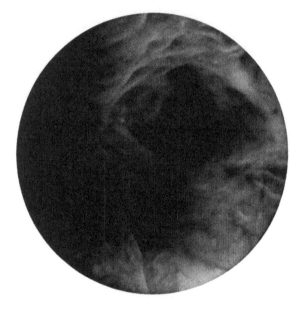

Fig. 17. Normal internal os of the uterus. Age 39. The somewhat irregular circle of the internal os of the uterus of a multiparous woman is distendable by a little oppression of the outer sleeve of hysteroscope

Fig. 18. Normal internal os of the uterus. Age 24. The narrow circular internal os of a nulliparous woman is so rigid as to require a Hegar dilator after paracervical anesthesia

6.2 Pathological Findings of the Cervix

6.2.1 Nabothian Cyst

One of the most frequent lesions is a round protrusion with white, pearl-like clusters. It is a cyst caused by occlusion of the glandular openings of the endocervix, the so-called nabothian cyst (Figs. 19, 20). During low-pressure fluid hysteroscopy, the *whitish*, stretched mucosal pattern with its plentiful fine vessels is appreciated.

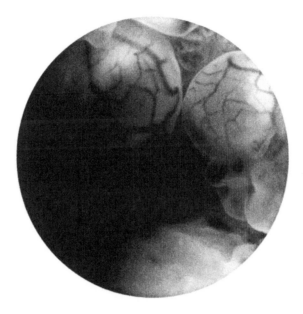

Fig. 19. Multiple nabothian cyst in the cervical canal. Age 42. Translucent, polypous projections developing from the cervical wall show a few hairy vessels on the surface

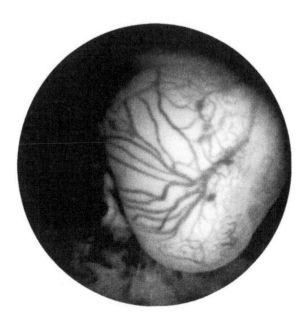

Fig. 20. Cystic polyp of the endocervix. Age 61. The polyp, which seems to have originated from a nabothian cyst, is *white* and translucent. The hairy aspects of the regularly branched vascular network are conspicuous

6.2.2 Endocervical Polyp

Endocervical polyps are often seen in the external os with the aid of a vaginal speculum. Occasionally these may disappear entirely in the cervical canal, causing abnormal bleeding. Endocervical polyps generally have a thin pedicle on which a lining of hairy, branched, vascular network can be seen (Figs. 21–24).

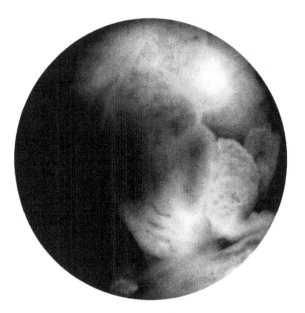

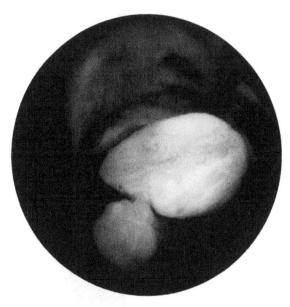

Fig. 21. Multiple polyps of the endocervix. Age 51. Tiny polyps developing from the posterior wall of the cervix caused slight postmenopausal bleeding

Fig. 22. Multiple polyps of the endocervix. Age 59. Two polyps hang from the upper cervical canal and appear *white-pink* in color. The atrophic surrounding endocervix shows a few crests

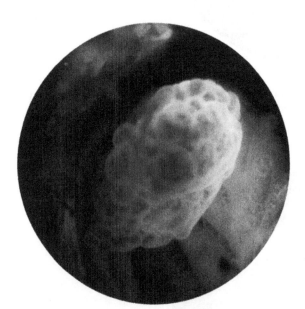

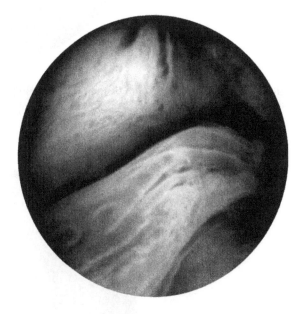

Fig. 23. Papillary endocervical polyp. Age 34. The polyp with a raspberry-shaped structure and *pink* vascularity can be seen in the core of each papilla

Fig. 24. Pedicle of endocervical polyp developing from the internal cervical os. Age 46. The thin pedicle is lined with some traces of the plica palmatae

6.2.3 Submucosal Cervical Leiomyoma

Cervical myoma bulging into the cervical canal is rare. It is a round protrusion with a wrinkled surface peculiar to that of the endocervical canal (Figs. 25, 26).

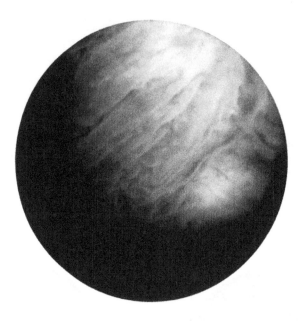

Fig. 25. Submucosal leiomyoma of the cervix. Age 32. The cervical canal is distorted by the nodule of leiomyoma bulging into the canal. The surface is covered with creased mucosa peculiar to the endocervix

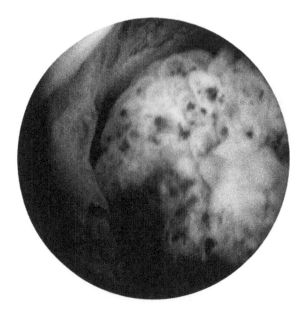

Fig. 26. Submucosal leiomyoma of the cervix. Age 31. The cervical canal is full of a hard, round tumor with papillary mucosa. It is necessary to differentiate this from papillomatous carcinoma

6.2.4 Chronic Cervicitis

Not infrequently, the endocervical mucosa with dilated vessels or plentiful small papillary projections is visible (Figs. 27, 28). Histology shows chronic cervicitis.

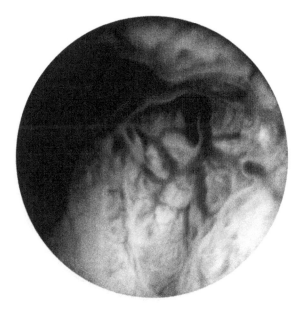

Fig. 27. Chronic cervicitis. Age 32. C.C.: Increased mucoserous discharge. Distended vessels around the stenotic internal os are regularly arranged. These vascularities seem to be caused by chronic inflammatory stimulation

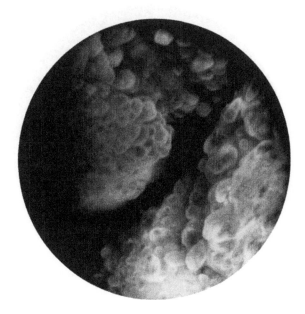

Fig. 28. Chronic cervicitis. Age 58. C.C.: Contact bleeding. Numerous papillary processes lying close together form a few cluster. It appears that they result from chronic irritation by infection

6.2.5 Cervical Synechia

In older women, the anterior and posterior walls of the isthmus occasionally may adhere to each other, especially in those patients who have undergone numerous D&C (Figs. 29–31). Complete occlusion of the isthmus, causing secondary amenorrhea with molimen, is rare (Figs. 32, 33a,b).

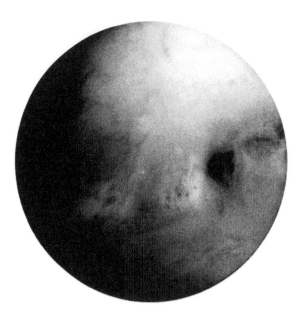

Fig. 29. Synechia of the internal os. Age 53. C.C.: Intermittent yellow discharge after menopause. The cervical canal is *whitish-yellow* in color and lined with a flat endocervix. Pale adhesion can be seen on both sides of a punctiform internal os. Pyorrhea cannot be seen because the canal has been irrigated beforehand

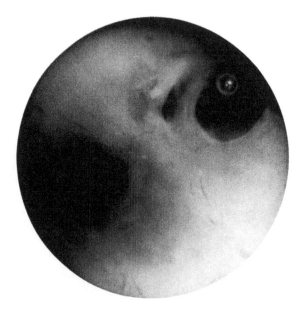

Fig. 30. Synechia of the internal os. Age 34. A bridgelike structure was found at the time of reexamination by hysteroscopy, 8 weeks after vaginal endometrial polypectomy. The internal os is divided into two holes by this synechia. The adhesion was easily torn off by pushing with the distal tip of the endoscope

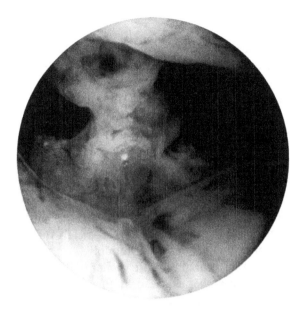

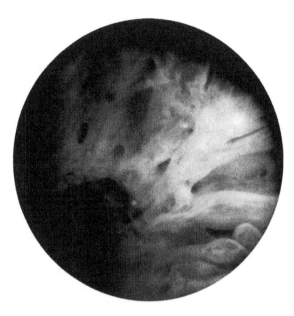

Fig. 31. Cervical synechia. Age 51. There is a bridgelike synechia on this side of the internal os. The patient had experienced D&C several times

Fig. 32. Complete occlusion of the internal os. Age 66. C.C.: Intermittent lower abdominal pain. The uterus was slightly swollen, with tenderness. Hysteroscopy could find only a trace of the internal os in the depth of the distended cervical canal. The lining is a mucosa with plicae and crypts peculiar to the endocervix. Cervical dilatation by Hegar dilator resulted in a drain of mucoserous fluid and disappearance of pain

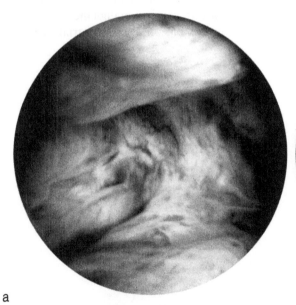

a

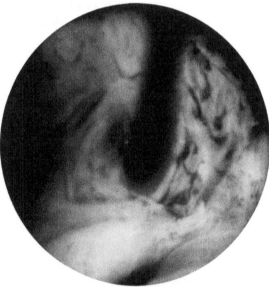

b

Fig. 33a,b. Complete occlusion of the internal os. Age 32. C.C.: Amenorrhea since her last delivery, 8 months previously, and periodic lower abdominal pain. Basal body temperature (BBT) showed a biphasic pattern. **a** The top of the cervical canal is closed with a filmy structure that appears translucent and pale. **b** As soon as

the tip of the sound broke through the membrane of the adhesion, *brown* fluid gushed out from the uterine cavity. The pain completely disappeared after a continuous drain of the fluid, and the patient's regular periods have since returned

6.2.6 Endocervical Malignancy

There are two types of intracervical malignancy: cervical carcinoma beyond the view of colposcopy (unsatisfactory colposcopy, UC) and cervical invasion of endomerial carcinoma. The latter is be described in a later chapter.

The squamocolumnar junction (SCJ) may be located within the endocervical canal in some older, particularly postmenopausal, women. In spite of abnormal Papanicolaou smears of cervical scraping samples, colposcopy may show a normal appearance of the endocervix. UC is to be alternated with hysteroscopy or endocervicoscopy. Hamou (1981) reported microhysteroscopic findings of neoplastic changes in the transformation zone, which is within the cervical canal. He confirmed that the instrument could identify neoplasia in this region, stained by blue ink in advance, just as accurately as Papanicolaou smears, and that microhysteroscopically directed conization obviated the need for blind diagnostic conization.

Hysteroscopic images of intracervical carcinoma are similar to the findings observed with a colposcope. They are characterized by the color, opacity, coarseness, and unevenness of the lining epithelia with abnormal vascularities. The appearance is sharply demarcated by application of acetic acid. As invasion progresses, the opaque white epithelium becomes more uneven and ragged with an increase in the irregular network of engorged, bizarre vessels as well as marked punctation (Figs. 34–37). Endocervical adenocarcinoma is not so frequent. It can be identified endoscopically as papillary or finely polypous projections with atypical vascularities (Figs. 38–41).

As invasion reaches deeper, ulceration and the accompanying atypical vessels become markedly conspicuous. Thus, hysteroscopy is valuable not only to detect intracervical carcinoma but also to confirm the diagnosis whenever a discrepancy between cytology and histology occurs. Another advantage of hysteroscopy for diagnosis of intracervical malignancy, as described later (pp. 106), is detection of cervical extension of endometrial carcinoma.

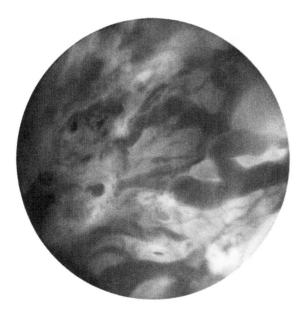

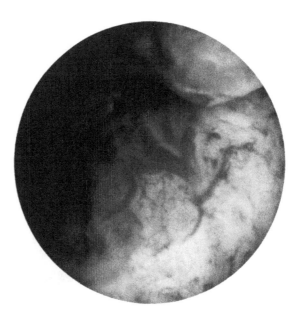

Fig. 34. Intracervical carcinoma (UC Ib). Age 50. Colposcopically, the squamocolumnar junction (SCJ) was invisible. Squamous cell carcinoma near the internal os shows uneven eminences on which surface bizarre branching vessels irregularly creep

Fig. 35. Intracervical carcinoma (UC Ib). Age 58. C.C.: Contact bleeding. Despite a class 5 Pap smear, the patient showed an unsatisfactory colposcopic (UC) finding. A hemispheric prominence with bizarre vascularity can be seen at 2 to 7 o'clock on this side of the internal os. Histology showed invasive squamous cell carcinoma

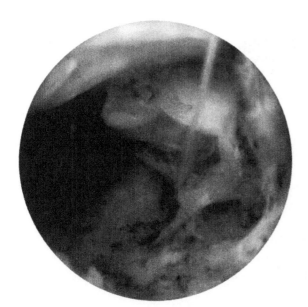

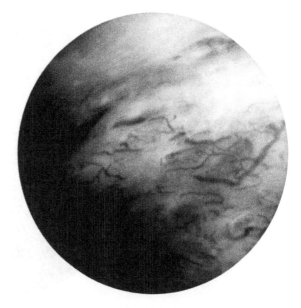

Fig. 36. Intracervical carcinoma (UC Ib). Age 59. This case also showed unsatisfactory colposcopy. Irregular projections are localized at 1 to 5 o'clock. Part of the lesions seem to turn into necrosis

Fig. 37. Intracervical carcinoma (UC IIb). Age 63. The SCJ can be seen at the depth of the external os. The left-lower part of the endocervical canal is unevenly elevated. Shaggy vascularity is a characteristic finding of malignancy

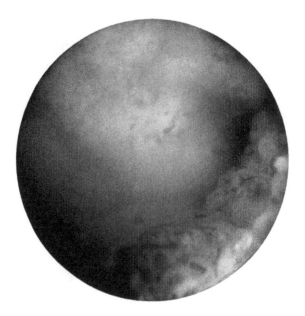

Fig. 38. Intracervical adenocarcinoma. Age 73. C.C.: Postmenopausal bleeding. The endocervical smear was suspected of malignancy, but colposcopy was unsatisfactory. Hysteroscopy revealed short papillary projections at the left-posterior part of the endocervix, which are sharply demarcated from the surrounding atrophic endocervix. This finding is evidence of adenocarcinoma

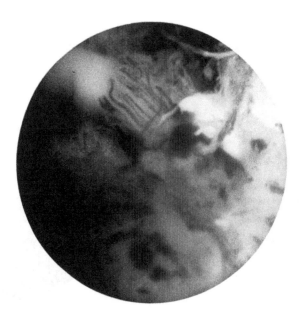

Fig. 39. Intracervical adenocarcinoma. Age 73. At 1 to 8 o'clock, irregular, ragged ulceration, partly with papillary projections, can be observed

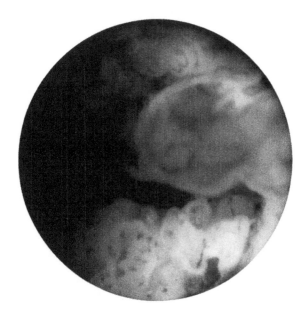

Fig. 40. Minimally invasive adenocarcinoma of the endocervix. Age 43. C.C.: Contact bleeding. Colposcopy showed normal finding. The lesion is made up partly of polypous and partly of papillary adenocarcinoma

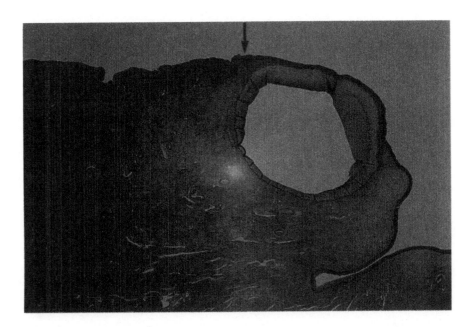

Fig. 41. Histology (longitudinal section of the cervix) of intracervical carcinoma. Age 58. The squamocolumnar junction (SCJ) has withdrawn into the cervical canal. The lesion of carcinoma is visible just above the SCJ (*arrow*)

7 The Uterine Body

As the hysteroscope is slowly advanced into the cervical canal under direct vision, the isthmus (the internal os), which is a flattened, narrowed circle, becomes clearer. The surface is smoother than that of the highly folded endocervix. In most multiparous women, the general rigid hysteroscope with an outer sleeve (7-mm OD) can be introduced through the isthmus without prior mechanical dilatation. In nulliparous or aged women, however, the cervical canal may have to be dilated to a diameter of 7 mm in advance, and then the outer sheath with an obturator is introduced beyond the level of the internal os. The obturator is removed and replaced with a hysteroscope. When the irrigating fluid returns clear, the flow is stopped by closing the drain valve and the uterine cavity is visualized in its totality. A detailed examination begins near the internal os and proceeds gradually upward to the fundus and the uterine cornua.

First of all, before the diagnosis of intrauterine abnormalities by using hysterocopy, it is absolutely necessary to be familiar with the normal images of hysteroscopy, especially its cyclic, gestational, and senile changes.

7.1 Normal Findings of the Uterine Cavity

7.1.1 Cyclic Changes in Reproductive Age

The first successful hysterocopy of cyclic changes of the endometrium in reproductive age was performed by Schroeder in 1934. Graphically presenting cyclic changes of the endometrium sketched by an artist, he stated that the endometrium immediately after menstruation was *yellowish-red* in color and could hardly be distinguished from the endocervix, but thereafter it became possible to roughly discriminate the phases of the menstrual cycle on hysteroscopy. Also, he described that in the secretory phase, the endometrium became thicker, protruded partly into the uterine cavity, and in the premenstrual phase it changed from *reddish* to *whitish* as the result of stromal edema, showing partial shedding was ready to take place. Nearly the same description was also given by Gribb in 1960. He found the correct identification rate for the proliferative phase was 80%, for the midcycle 75%, and for the secretory phase 72%.

Certainly our experience also admits that it is possible to distinguish more detailed findings of each phase of the menstrual cycle. The identification is made on the basis of thickness of the endometrium, undulations and folds of the lining, the indentation of the gland opening, changes in color from stromal edema, vasculature, and so on.

7.1.1.1 Menstrual Phase

The chance that hysteroscopy will be used to view the precise moment of onset of bleeding is very small. On the surface of the involutional endometrium immediately before menstruation, tiny blood blebs may extrude up and down (Figs. 42, 43). These become inflated and burst open in an instance that is not yet endometrial shedding. At the time the patient is aware of the onset of menstruation, hysteroscopy can be used to see no more than the uterine cavity in which the endometrium has already shed. Endometrial shedding in menstruation appears to take place throughout the uterine cavity, unlike dysfunctional uterine bleeding (Fig. 44). At first, water hysteroscopy during menstruation may be often interrupted to get a clear view because the rinsing fluid mixes with blood. As irrigation is patiently done, the rinsing fluid gradually becomes clear and makes it possible to get a clear view. The denuded lining in the uterine cavity appears ragged, exposing fresh wounds. As the rinsing fluid flow is stopped by closing the drain valve, blood flow gushing through creeks of the stripped stumps can be seen (Figs. 45, 46).

As menstruation progresses, the surface of the uterine cavity gradually becomes flattened, leaving crowded ciliary processes that seem to be the stumps of broken blood vessels and glands. Small blood spots also lie scattered about (Figs. 47–49).

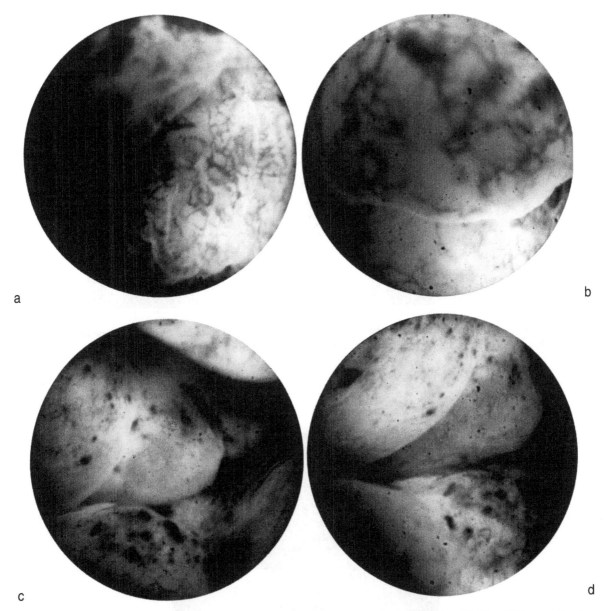

a

b

c

d

Fig. 42. Involutional late secretory endometrium immediately before menstruation. Age 30. Blood blisters of various sizes appear at various places on the surface of the endometrium

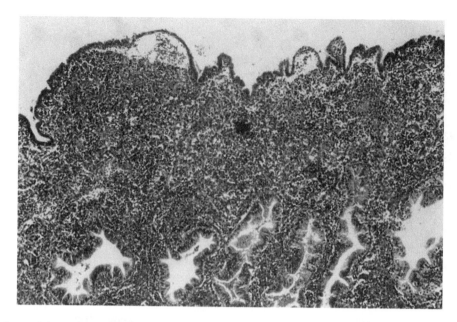

Fig. 43. Histology of the endometrium at the time when menstruation is just about to begin. A few microhematomas just under the lining epithelium and stromal bleeding are suggestive of the onset of menstruation

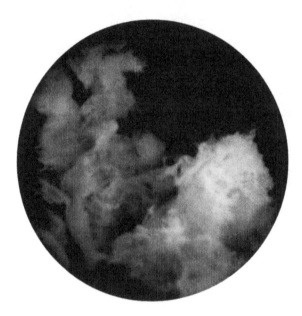

Fig. 44. Menstruating uterine cavity (day 2 of the cycle). Age 39. Although shedding of the endometrium occurs uniformly all over, the villous stumps remain

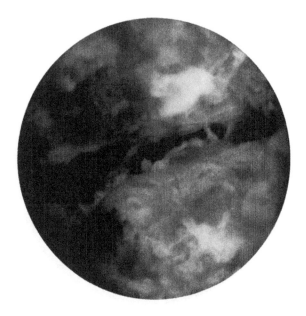

Fig. 45. Menstruating uterine cavity (day 3 of the cycle). Age 38. Shedding has nearly ended, but the surface is still uneven

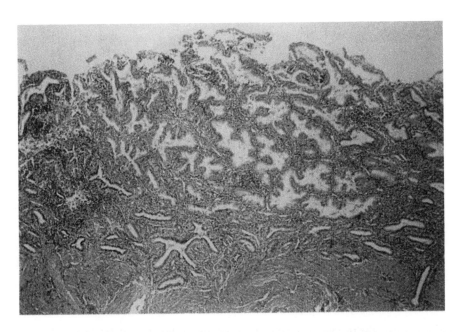

Fig. 46. Menstruating endometrium (day 1 of the cycle). Age 28. The apical layer of the late secretory endometrium is exfoliated

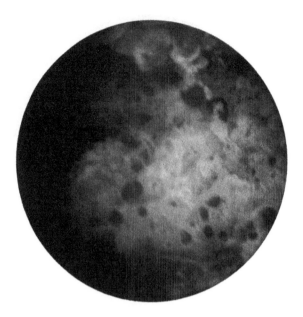

Fig. 47. The uterine cavity in the regenerative phase (day 6 of the cycle). Age 27. The surface is still shaggy with stumps of blood vessels and glands and has fine spotted ecchymoses

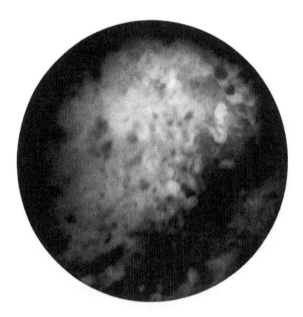

Fig. 48. The uterine cavity in the regenerative phase (day 6 of the cycle). Age 30. Pilelike projections of the stumps of blood vessels and glands are still conspicuous although menstrual bleeding has stopped

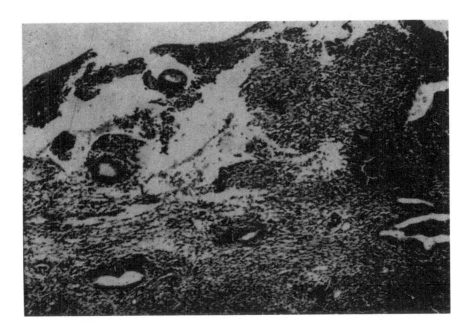

Fig. 49. Menstruating endometrium (day 4 of the cycle). Age 34. The endometrium almost exfoliates, leaving a denuded surface. The small particles of the upper layer are being cast off

7.1.1.2 Regenerative Phase

As menstrual bleeding stops (on the fifth to sixth day of the cycle), the bare surface is completely covered with a regenerated endometrium, leaving a few blood spots (Fig. 50). The gently undulating surface looks velvety and *yellowish-red*. Few blood vessels are discernible, although tiny blood spots may remain here and there (Figs. 51, 52). This phase is most suitable for hysteroscopic confirmation of intrauterine abnormalities revealed by imaging techniques, because the uterine cavity is lined by the thinnest endometrium and is most liable to dilate even under low rinsing water pressure of any time in the menstrual cycle.

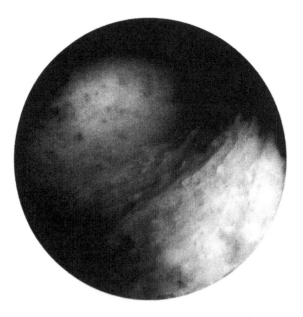

Fig. 50. The uterine cavity in the early proliferative phase (day 8 of the cycle). Age 40. The uterine cavity is completely covered with the renewed endometrium, although a few bleeding spots remain. Because the lining is thin and smooth and the uterus is easy to dilate even under a lower pressure of irrigating fluid, this phase provides the best opportunity for hysteroscopic examination of intrauterine abnormalities

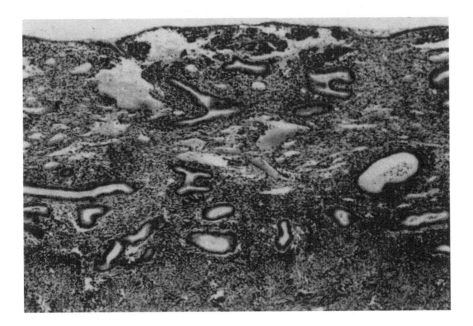

Fig. 51. Regenerative endometrium (day 6 of the cycle). Age 34. The surface is almost lined with a renewed endometrium. Note dilated lymph vessels in the stroma

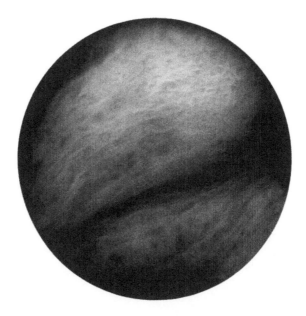

Fig. 52. The uterine cavity in the midproliferative phase. Age 45. As the cycle progresses, the endometrium is thickened, showing fine wrinkles on the surface, and is *yellowish-red* in color

7.1.1.3 Midproliferative Phase

As the endometrium gradually thickens, the surface increases its gentle undulations and appears livid in color. Glandular openings and vascularity are not conspicuous yet (Figs. 53–55).

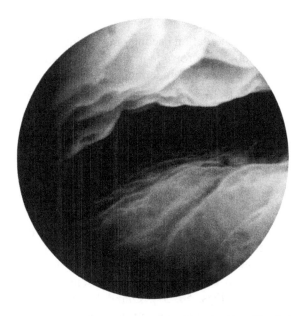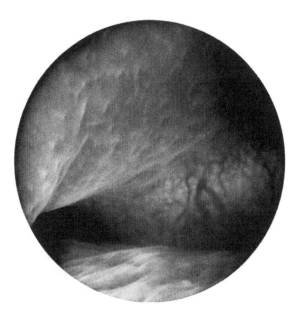

Fig. 53. The uterine cavity in midcycle (day 13 of the cycle). Age 31. Deep wrinkles are characteristic. Crypts can be seen corresponding with the glandular opening

Fig. 54. The uterine cavity in midcycle (day 14 of the cycle). Age 44. Hollowed glandular openings are regularly distributed. Subepithelial vessels are indistinct except for those of the fundal portion

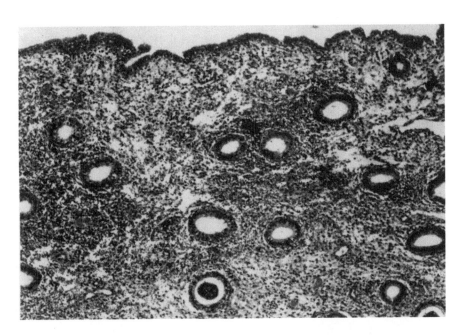

Fig. 55. Midproliferative endometrium (day 9 of the cycle). Age 27. The endometrium is thin, the glands are small and straight, and the stroma is compact. The surface is rather smooth

7.1.1.4 Midcycle

As the cycle progresses, the surface undulation becomes increasingly remarkable. Occasionally the endometrium may protrude in a moundlike state into the uterine cavity, with multiple punctuated indentations of the glandular openings. The tense surface of each projection is deeply *livid* in color in spite of the undistinguishable vascularity. As the uterine cavity distends with a rise of rinsing water pressure, these protrusions and color gradually fade. In the midcycle, which is dominant in estrogen levels, panoramic hysteroscopy is most difficult to perform because of thickening of the endometrium and the increasing muscle contractility.

7.1.1.5 Secretory Phase

Hysteroscopy is difficult to use to distinguish the midcycle and the early secretory phase. The lining endometrium in the midsecretory phase is thick and polypous, and appears *yellow-red* and *translucent* because of stromal edema. Hysteroscopy can be used to view clearly shaggy vascular patterns throughout the translucent stroma (Figs. 56, 57). Glandular openings no longer appear on the stretched surface of polypous projections.

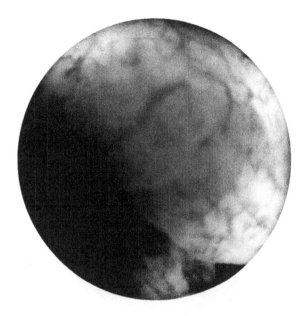

Fig. 56. The uterine cavity in the midsecretory phase (day 21 of the cycle). Age 38. As polypoid protrusions of the endometrium are markedly engorged, gland openings become indistinct. The edematous stroma becomes so translucent that the subepithelial vascular network is prominent

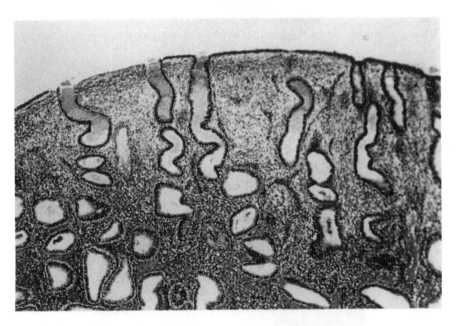

Fig. 57. Midsecretory endometrium (day 20 of the cycle). Age 28. Moderately tortuous glands with definite secretion are arranged regularly toward the surface. Many small vessels are distributed in the markedly edematous stroma

7.1.1.6 Involutional Phase

If ovum implantation does not occur, the endometrium begins to shrink because of a decrease of stromal edema and looks less *translucent* and *red-yellow* in color. Hysteroscopy can be used to see the polypoid endometrium with an uneven surface, which loses tonus and wrinkles. The hairy, shaggy aspect of the vascular network is still visible (Figs. 58–60). Immediately before the onset of menstruation, tiny blood spots begin to appear, but the endometrium does not desquamate yet (Figs. 61, 62).

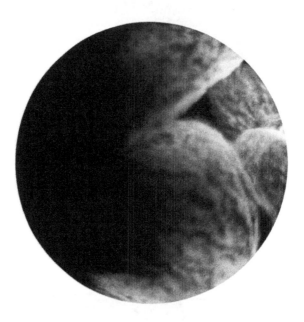

Fig. 58. The uterine cavity in the late secretory phase (day 26 of the cycle). Age 29. As stromal edema has nearly receded, the mucosal protrusions are rather withered, leaving the wrinkled surface

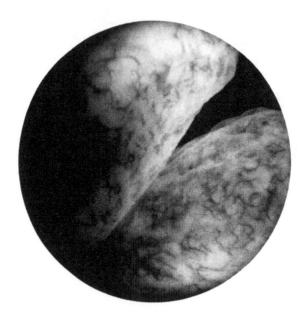

Fig. 59. The uterine cavity in the late secretory phase (day 27 of the cycle). Age 29. As involution advances, engorged polypoid protrusions wither much more. Stromal edema and visible vessels decrease, and superficial wrinkles increase

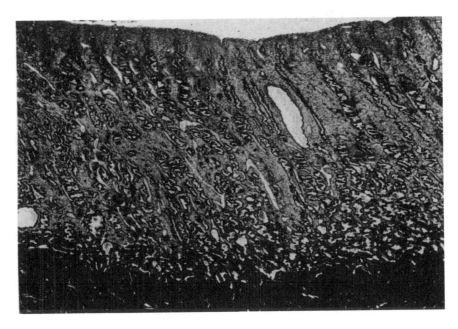

Fig. 60. Late secretory endometrium (day 25 of the cycle). Age 42. Tortuous glands grow close together in the stroma with rather shrinking edema

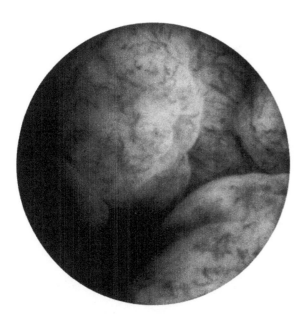

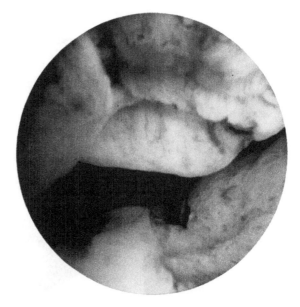

Fig. 61. The uterine cavity just before menstruation. Age 29. Polypoid projections of the endometrium appear somewhat *opaque*, and subepithelial vessels also decrease

Fig. 62. The uterine cavity just before menstruation (day 29 of the cycle). Age 40. Polypoid projections of the endometrium are rather *opaque*. Subepithelial blood vessels are indiscernible, but tiny blood spots may appear here and there

7.1.2 Early Pregnancy

Because hysteroscopic examination is usually contraindicated in early intrauterine pregnancy, it is very rare for hysteroscopy to be used to view early pregnancy. A sophisticated version of the now-available hysteroscope is considered to be able to view very early nidation, but we, unfortunately, have not had such an opportunity yet. The endometrial part, the decidua capsularis, embracing an embryo in the fifth to seventh week of gestation, shows a hemispheric elevation that on the surface looks *ruddy*. The vascular network on it is unclear. The endometrium around the gestational part, the parietal decidua, is thicker and smoother than that in the late secretory endometrium, because the uterine cavity not only distends with the progress of pregnancy but also is liable to dilate even by lower pressure of the rinsing fluid. The glandular openings surrounded by a fine capillary network dilate remarkably, producing a cribriform pattern peculiar to decidualization of the endometrium (Figs. 63–66). As pregnancy progresses, the capsular decidua becomes thin and pale. Its opacity, however, does not permit viewing the fetus through the membrane.

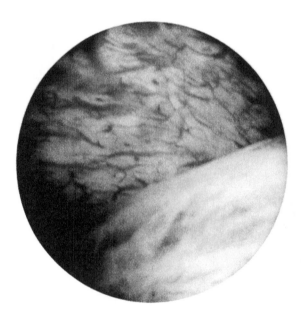

Fig. 63. The uterine cavity in early pregnancy (week 7 of gestation). Age 31. In the *lower half*, the capsular decidua, which hemispherically protrudes into the cavity, appears rather faded, while in the *upper half*, the parietal decidua is abundant in the vascular network

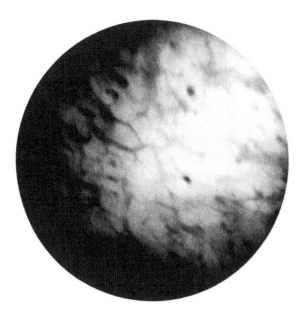 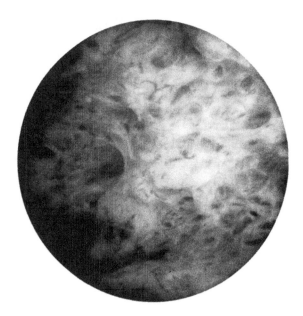

Fig. 64. The uterine cavity in early pregnancy (week 7 of gestation). Age 31. A typical parietal decidua in early pregnancy is characterized by tangled vascularity surrounding dilated glandular openings

Fig. 65. The uterine cavity in early pregnancy (week 8 of gestation). Age 32. Crater-like dilatation of the glandular opening is marked in a part saved from the pressure of the capsular decidua. The dilated openings gather and form a cribriform pattern of the decidua

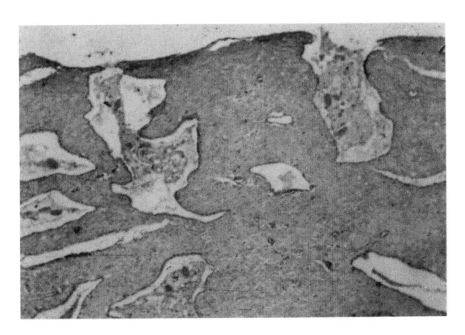

Fig. 66. Decidua in early pregnancy (week 7 of gestation). Age 31. In the thickened parietal decidua, dilated glands are sparse and filled with a lot of secretion. The secretion flows from the opening to the surface

7.1.3 Postmenopause

Characteristics of a postmenopausal uterus are involution of the uterine body and thinning of the endometrium with no cyclic change. The uterine cavity is easily dilated, even by using low-pressure rinsing fluid. The endometrium is thin, flat, and *yellowish-white* throughout the uterine cavity. No glandular openings or vascular network is visible (Figs. 67–69). Occasionally thin-walled cystic glands are derived from occlusion of the glandular openings, simulating nabothian cysts of the cervix.

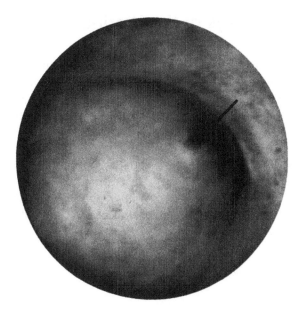

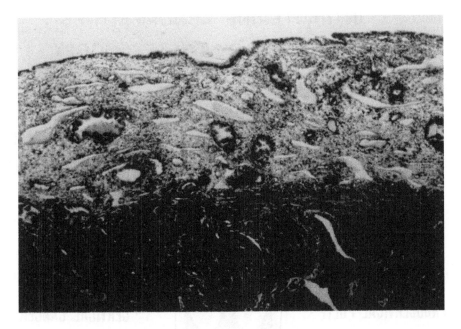

Fig. 67. The senile uterine cavity (10 years after menopause). Age 60. The senile uterus is easy to distend even by a slight pressure of irrigating fluid. The surface is flattened and appears *pinkish-yellow* because the subepithelial blood vessels are poor. The left tubal ostium looks like a small spot (*arrow*)

Fig. 68. A bird's-eye view of senile uterine cavity (7 years after menopause). Age 56. The whole uterine cavity is lined by thin endometrium. This photography commands a complete view of the uterine cavity: the fundus, bilateral cornua, and side walls

Fig. 69. Senile atrophic endometrium (16 years after menopause). Age 65. The thin senile endometrium is so atrophic that the functional layer is indistinguishable from the basal one. The gland with low cuboidal epithelium becomes very sparse

7.2 Pathological Findings of the Uterine Cavity

Essentially, hysteroscopy is performed just after menstruation has completely terminated to obtain accurate findings without the obstacles of blood and debris. When the origin of abnormal bleeding has to be elucidated, however, hysteroscopy should be done at any time during the bleeding. Examination begins near the internal os and proceeds gradually upward to the uterine fundus and the uterine cornua. According to the findings peculiar to intrauterine abnormalities, the uterine cavity, differing from the normal surrounding endometrium, is characterized by roughness, ulceration, elevation, or protrusion of the surface, bleeding spots, and vascular pattern (Fig. 70). Suspect lesions can be biopsied with special forceps under visual control.

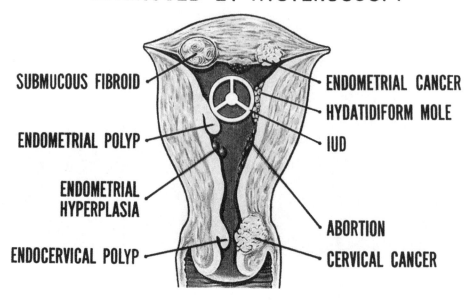

INTRAUTERINE ABNORMALITIES DIAGNOSED BY HYSTEROSCOPY

SUBMUCOUS FIBROID

ENDOMETRIAL POLYP

ENDOMETRIAL HYPERPLASIA

ENDOCERVICAL POLYP

ENDOMETRIAL CANCER

HYDATIDIFORM MOLE

IUD

ABORTION

CERVICAL CANCER

Fig. 70. Scheme of organic lesions causing abnormal uterine bleeding. Although these endometrial pathologies do not always induce abnormal bleeding, hysteroscopy is a good way to check the source of bleeding

7.2.1 Dysfunctional Uterine Bleeding

Abnormal uterine bleeding is one of the most common symptoms even in patients of reproductive age as well as in premenopausal or postmenopausal women. Hysteroscopy has become the most useful accurate method to evaluate whether bleeding is caused by organic lesions or dysfunctional disorders. The term dysfunctional uterine bleeding is often used in the clinical diagnosis for abnormal uterine bleeding originating from no organic lesion in the uterine cavity, although its concept is not strictly justified yet. In this chapter, it is defined as "abnormal bleeding from the endometrium, except for menstrual bleeding, in the absence of gross anatomic changes, for example, pregnancy, inflammation, neoplasm, chemical or mechanical irritation, and so on." Dysfunctional uterine bleeding can occur from the endometrium of each phase of the menstrual cycle. Therefore, the hysteroscopic view presents a picture similar to that of a variant of the normal endometrium.

First of all, before hysteroscopy, systemic diseases causing abnormal bleeding should be excluded by physical and laboratory examination. Next, endoscopists must discriminate organic lesions, although they do not always cause abnormal bleeding, and confirm that the bleeding originates from the dysfunctioning endometrium. Additionally, a hysteroscopic diagnosis of dysfunctional bleeding has to be made under the considerations of the process, duration, and amount of bleeding, the time relationship to menstruation, and hormone therapy.

7.2.1.1 Prolonged Menstruation

It may occasionally occur that menstruation continues for longer than 7 days and is accompanied by increased loss of blood (menorrhagia). In such cases, hysteroscopy can often sight bleeding as coming from still-unshed secretory endometrium; it seems that prolonged menstruation depends on irregular shedding of the endometrium because of luteal persistence for any reason. In most cases, the lining is almost completely sloughed, leaving only a few fragments of the secretory endometrium (Fig. 71), and in some cases, the greater part of the secretory endometrium may remain (Fig. 72). When abnormal bleeding starts some time before expected menstruation, there may appear to be a lot of fine thrombi on the surface of the unshed secretory endometrium (Fig. 73). Judging from what the endometrium has shown, the appearance so closly resembling a decidua in pregnancy, the bleeding seems to have resulted from subclinical abortion without any obvious sign of pregnancy (Fig. 74). As bleeding by irregular shedding of the endometrium is prolonged, the secretory endometrium is gradually replaced with the proliferative tissue (Figs. 75, 76).

Another prolonged menstruation, which spouts from a crack in the proliferative endometrium, may be often excessive, so-called anovulatory menstruation. Although this is different in duration of bleeding, part of the proliferative endometrium is left without complete sloughing, unlike normal menstruation. The unstripped endometrial lining is somewhat shrunk and *livid* in color (Figs. 77–80). The stripped endometrial lining is ciliarily thicker than the regenerative one after menstruation (Fig. 81), and multiple stumps of broken glands and vessels quivering in the rinsing fluid can be seen on hysteroscopy (Figs. 82, 83). This appearance is indicative of the violent rise and fall of hyperestrogenic states so that most of the proliferative endometrium remains unstripped. It is appreciated that the most reasonable treatment is to induce ovulation after withdrawal bleeding by estrogen-progesterone medication.

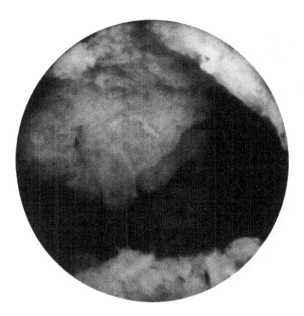

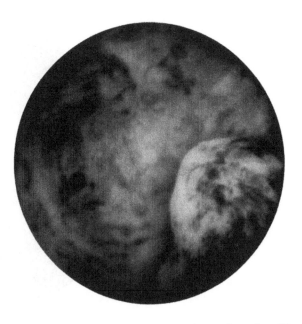

Fig. 71. Irregular shedding of the endometrium. Age 43. C.C.: Prolonged menstruation for 9 days. The secretory endometrium remains

Fig. 72. Irregular shedding of the endometrium. Age 35. C.C.: Prolonged menstruation for 10 days. Almost all the endometrium is sloughed, leaving a tiny part of the secretory polypous endometrium

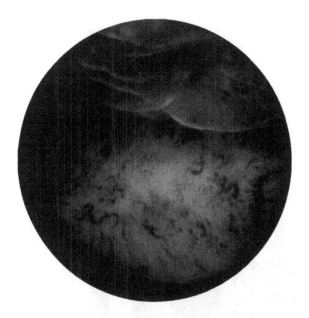

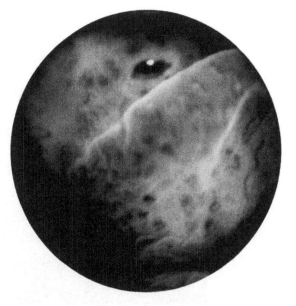

Fig. 73. Irregular shedding of the endometrium. Age 34. C.C.: Prolonged menstruation for 12 days. The patient's cycle (25-day interval) became a little shorter than usual, followed by menstruation for 12 days. On the surface of the unsloughed endometrium are many spiral thrombi

Fig. 74. Irregular shedding of the endometrium. Age 36. C.C.: Slight continuous bleeding just after menstruation that was shorter than usual. The greater part of the unshed endometrium shows a decidua-like appearance reminiscent of subclinical abortion. Punctate microthrombi on the surface, *brown* in color, are impressive

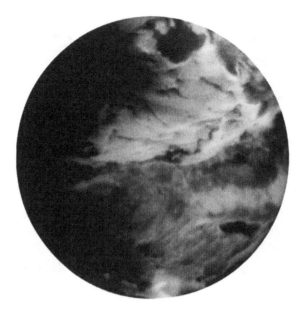

Fig. 75. Irregular shedding of the endometrium. Age 43. C.C.: Menstruation prolonged for 9 days. Although the endometrium is incompletely sloughed, renewal of the endometrium is going to begin (*bottom*)

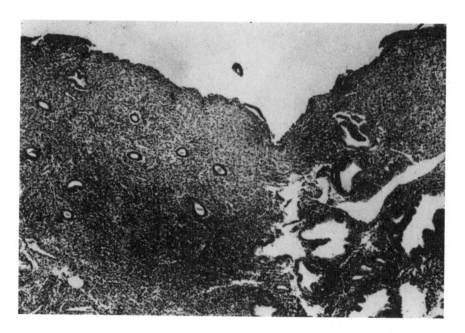

Fig. 76. Histology of coexistence of the secretory and proliferative endometrium in a case of irregular shedding. Age 46. The secretory endometrium on the *right side* contrasts with the proliferative one with sparse glands and compact stroma on the *left*

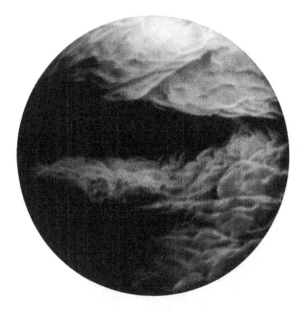

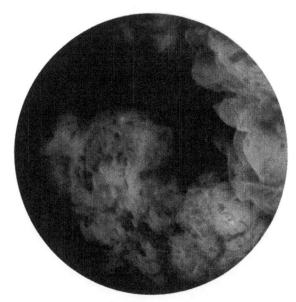

Fig. 77. Anovulatory menstruation. Age 27. C.C.: Anovulation. Although the patient wishes to bear a child, her BBT chart shows a low monophasic pattern. Bleeding began on day 30 of the cycle, and continued for 7 days. The photograph was taken on the first day of the bleeding. It looks exactly like the late proliferative endometrium without any collapse

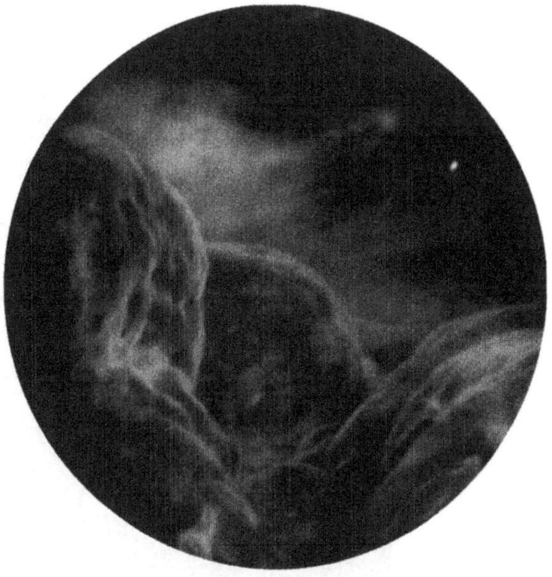

Fig. 78. Anovulatory menstruation. Age 36. C.C.: Wish for childbearing and hypomenorrhea. Her BBT chart shows a low monophasic pattern. The endometrium, although on the third day of the cycle, is hardly shed, like that of midcycle bleeding, maintaining a late proliferative appearance

Fig. 79. Anovulatory menstruation. Age 20. C.C.: Prolonged menstruation. Prolonged but intermittent bleeding may occur in a patient with a monophasic cycle. She complained of slight bleeding without medical treatment for about 3 months. Incompletely sloughed proliferative endometrium is retained on the whole surface of the uterine cavity

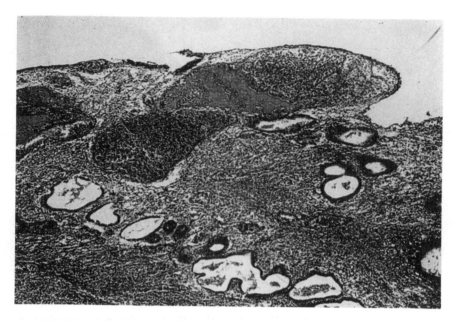

Fig. 80. Histology of the endometrium of anovulatory bleeding for a long time. Age 28. Irregularly shaped glands are sporadic. The stroma, with many spiral arteries, is remarkably infiltrated by red blood cells and platelets and partly holds small hematomas

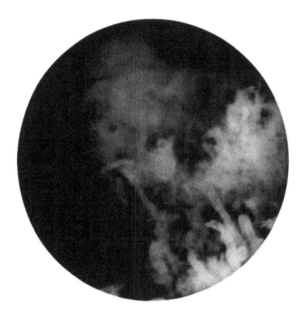

Fig. 81. Dysfunctional bleeding. Age 42. C.C.: Prolonged menstruation. This photograph was taken on day 21 after the onset of bleeding. The endometrium is almost shed, in part leaving villous projections unlike normal menstruation

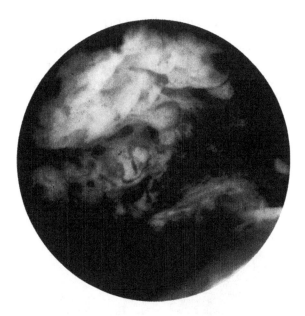

Fig. 82. Prolonged anovulatory bleeding. Age 28. C.C.: Abnormal bleeding that continued more than 14 days. The endometrium began to regenerate before complete desquamation

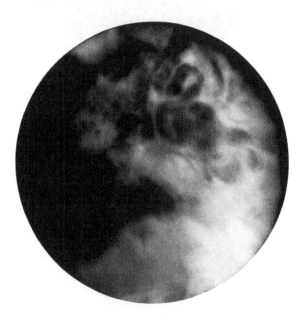

Fig. 83. Prolonged anovulatory bleeding. Age 47. C.C.: Abnormal bleeding that continued for 11 days. The endometrium is incompletely sloughed, leaving some spiral arteries filled with fresh thrombus

7.2.1.2 Midcycle Bleeding

Midcycle blood flow occurs from the proliferative endometrium during the preovulatory phase with a small fluctuation of estrogen. The small amount of the bleeding suggests that it is a breakthrough bleeding without endometrial shedding (Fig. 84).

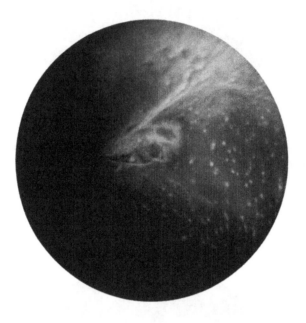

Fig. 84. Midcycle bleeding. Age 28. C.C.: Spotting at midcycle. Well-developed endometrium does not show shedding although so engorged

7.2.1.3 Abnormal Bleeding in the Secretory Phase

Abnormal bleeding during the late secretory phase may be rarely seen as premenstrual spotting (Figs. 85–87). It may occasionally occur while taking contraceptive pills and in pseudopregnancy therapy (as described in the next section). In most of these cases the endometrial lining retains the feature of the secretory endometrium without desquamation, although the surface is often dotted with tiny blood spots.

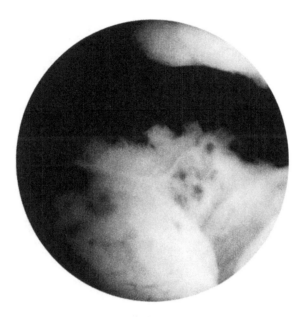

Fig. 85. Premenstrual spotting. Age 27. The late secretory endometrium on day 25 of the cycle, which is *whitish* in color and has receded vascularity, does not show shedding yet, but small blood spots appear slightly elevated on the surface

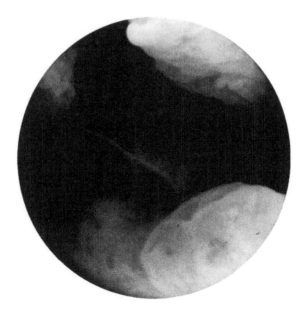

Fig. 86. Premenstrual spotting. Age 31. In part (*lower left*) of the endometrium on day 4 before the estimated period, subepithelial blood spots can be seen

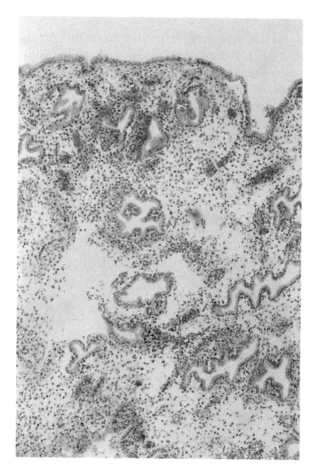

Fig. 87. Late secretory endometrium with premenstrual spotting. Age 25. On day 3 before the expected period, small ecchymoses and red blood cell infiltration appear in the stroma

7.2.2 Iatrogenic Bleeding During Long-Term Hormone Therapy

We often observe abnormal bleeding from the endometrium during long-term hormone treatment of menopause syndrome, endometriosis, atypical hyperplasia of the endometrium and breast cancer. The main hormones used are contraceptive pills (pseudopregnancy therapy and hormone replacement therapy), danazol, gonadotropin-releasing hormone (GnRH) analogue, and tamoxifen. Occasionally in the course of administration of these synthetic hormones, unexpected iatrogenic bleeding may occur. If a combined estrogen-progestogen pill is consecutively administered, the endometrium grows thick for the first several weeks (Fig. 88), showing decidua-like alteration. Sooner or later, however, its thickening somewhat recedes.

The uterine cavity is easy to distend by low-pressure rinsing fluid because of reduced contractility of the uterine wall. The lining epithelium becomes rather thin, and has a wrinkled surface with a remarkable dilated vascular network so as to confuse it with endometrial malignancy (Fig. 89). Bleeding occurs from a tear in the vessels (Fig. 90). As danazol suppresses the growth of the endometrium from the beginning, the uterine cavity looks like that in the midproliferative phase (Fig. 91). If bleeding occurs, although sometimes much and sometimes little, slightly elevated blood spots can be seen here and there on hysteroscopy (Fig. 92). GnRH agonist also, although this medication temporarily makes the endometrium thick because of temporary flare-up of estrogen at the early stage of the medication, restrains its growth because of continued hypoestrogenicity (Fig. 93). If there is any bleeding, tiny ecchymoses can be observed (Fig. 94).

Second-grade amenorrhea caused by severe ovarian dysfunction also provides endometrial hypoplasia, which shows a thin mucosa but a high vascular pattern unlike senile atrophic endometrium (Fig. 95). Tamoxifen, one of the antiestrogenic agents, is often used as an adjuvant hormone therapy after breast carcinoma operations; however, it may cause abnormal uterine bleeding during continued medication. The endometrium looks like that during danazol treatment (Fig. 96). Follow-up studies by medical treatment of atypical hyperplasia of the endometrium, using medroxyprogesterone acetate (MPA), are described in the next section.

Recently, hormone replacement therapy (HRT) has been popularly used for perimenopausal or postmenopausal women suffering from the more distressing symptoms. To avoid endometrial hyperplasia and abnormal bleeding associated with unopposed estrogen stimulation in HRT, current HRT tends to use a combination of minimal doses of estrogen and progestogen.

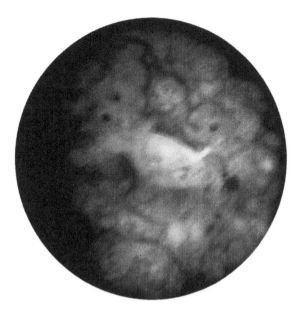

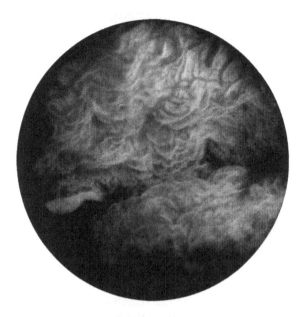

Fig. 88. The uterine cavity during pseudopregnancy therapy (day 45 of E-P pill medication). Age 45. C.C.: Dysmenorrhea. The patient has taken continuously a pill containing 5 mg of norethisterone and 0.05 mg of mestranol for 45 days for the purpose of medical treatment of endometriosis. The endometrium is thinner than that of normal pregnancy; however, distended glandular openings surrounded by thin vessels are suggestive of decidualization of the endometrium

Fig. 89. The uterine cavity during long-term pseudopregnancy therapy (week 25 of Norluten D medication). Age 37. Although the endometrium is thin, the surface shows fine crinkles with crooked vessels just like papillomatous carcinoma of the endometrium

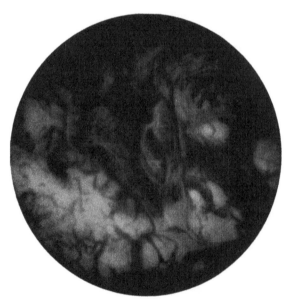

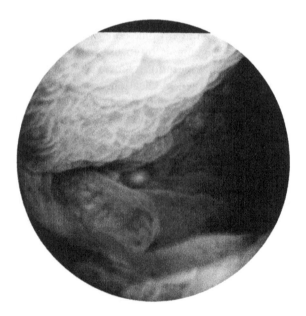

Fig. 90. Abnormal bleeding during pseudopregnancy therapy (week 27 of Norluten D medication). Age 42. C.C.: Spotting during pseudopregnancy therapy. When the patient had taken Norluten D for 20 weeks consecutively to relieve severe pain caused by endometriosis, she was aware of abnormal spotting. On the surface of the thin endometrium, a bristle vascular network is observed in bold relief against the uterine cavity. It seems that bleeding was caused by a break of these vessels. The glandular ostia are already inconspicuous

Fig. 91. The uterine cavity during continuous danazol therapy (week 17 of danazol medication, 400 mg per day). Age 44. C.C.: Dysmenorrhea. The endometrium is thin; however, the surface shows fine wrinkles like early secretory endometrium. No vascular network can be seen

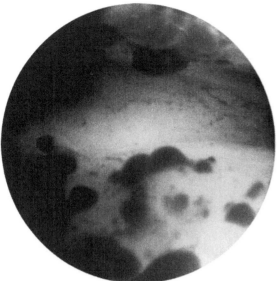

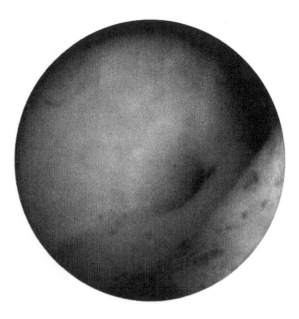

Fig. 92. Abnormal bleeding during danazol therapy (week 7 of danazol medication, 400 mg per day). Age 37. C.C.: Menses-like bleeding during danazol treatment. Fairly untoward bleeding began in week 6 of danazol medication. The surface of the thin endometrium is flattened and anemic. Slightly inflated blood spots are interspersed

Fig. 93. The uterine cavity during Buserelin medication (week 23 of Buserelin medication, 900 μg per day). Age 36. C.C.: Wish for childbearing and pelvic pain. Thin lining mucosa looks like senile atrophy of the endometrium. No glandular opening and vessel are visible

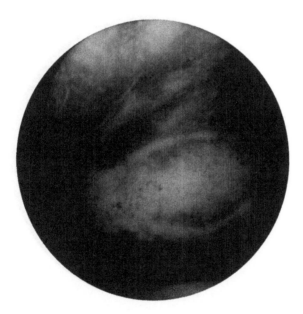

Fig. 94. Spotting during Buserelin therapy (day 41 of Buserelin medication, 900 μg per day). Age 36. The endometrium continued to thin but is studded by a few ecchymoses

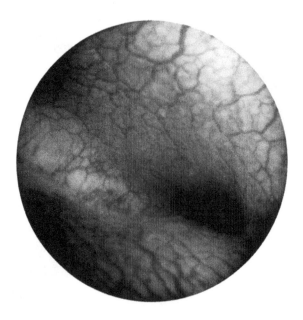

Fig. 95. The uterine cavity in a case of second-grade amenorrhea (35 pg/ml serum estradiol). Age 39. C.C.: Secondary amenorrhea. Although the endometrium is thin, subepithelial vessels are preserved

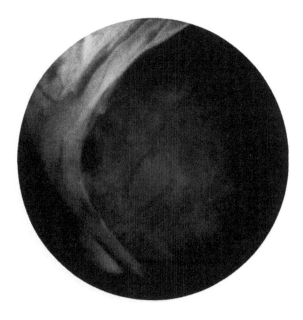

Fig. 96. Spotting during tamoxifen therapy (day 29 of tamoxifen medication, 30 mg per day). Age 67. C.C.: Spotting during adjuvant tamoxifen therapy after a radical operation for breast cancer. The patient was operated on for breast cancer 4 months previously. After about 80 days of tamoxifen administration, she noticed vaginal spotting. The thin endometrium with subepithelial angiectasis is partly shed, and a few blood spots are dotted

7.2.3 Endometrial Hyperplasia

Endometrial hyperplasia has been histologically divided into three patterns: cystic glandular hyperplasia, adenomatous hyperplasia, and atypical hyperplasia. It is unsuitable, however, to apply this histological classification of hyperplasia wholly to hysteroscopy. Especially, cystic glandular hyperplasia in histology is thought of a representative of low-risk hyperplasia. Hysteroscopic diagnosis of endometrial hyperplasia is determined by the thickness, color, vasculature, unevenness, and plasticity of the endometrium. So, from both the clinical and hysteroscopic standpoints, endometrial hyperplasia is properly divided into two criteria, a low-risk and high-risk category (Mencaglia and Perino 1989); furthermore, low-risk hyperplasia is classified into simple, polypoid (focal), and cystic hyperplasia, and high-risk hyperplasia is divided into adenomatous and atypical. The slower but continual ablation of hyperplastic endometrium prolongs abnormal bleeding, and the more complex the hysteroscopic aspect becomes because of collapse of the original features of the lesion on one hand and of renewal of the endometrium on the other. Thus, hysteroscopic diagnosis in principle is aimed at the lesion saved from ablation.

7.2.3.1 Low-Risk Endometrial Hyperplasia

The gross appearance of benign endometrial hyperplasia associated with a continuous hyperestrogenic state is close to that of the normal endometrium at the end of the late proliferative phase when the mucosa reaches its peak of thickness.

Simple hyperplasia, which clinically causes a kind of "dysfunctional uterine bleeding" in a broad sense, is closely similar to the endometrium in the preovulatory phase in regards to color, unevenness, and plasticity. The highly increased thickness of the mucosa is assessed by means of pressure by the tip of the hysteroscope, resulting in a dent. The well-developed endometrium appears *livid* in color, sparse in vascularity, and deep in indentation of the glandular opening (Figs. 97, 98). As the bleeding is prolonged, mucosal ablation occurs in disorderly fashion here and there, leaving behind many unsloughed endometrial fragments, rather thick stumps of vessels and glands, unlike normal menstruation (Figs. 99–101). Blood spouts from the splits of the mucosa and vascular stumps. Eventually it is fairly difficult to discriminate simple endometrial hyperplasia from the continually proliferating endomerium associated with common dysfunctional bleeding.

The hysteroscopic diagnosis of focal hyperplasia is easily made because its outgrowth displays the exact image objectively. The polypous or moundlike projections may be either solitary or multiple and do not always produce abnormal bleeding (Figs. 102–104). If any, bleeding occurs from the tip of the projection without tissue collapse. The appearance of each projection on hysteroscopy is similar to that of simple endometrial hyperplasia (Figs. 105–108).

In cystic endometrial hyperplasia, on histology the gland is uniformly dilated and enlarged, accounting for the characteristic "Swiss cheese" pattern. The hysteroscopic aspect of cystic endometrial hyperplasia cannot, however, often discern the cystic relief raised on the surface because the cystic gland is deeply concealed in the stroma, but only shows the feature in a fashion analogous to simple endometrial hyperplasia (Fig. 109).

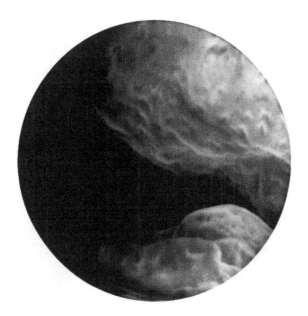

Fig. 97. Simple hyperplasia of the endometrium. Age 51. C.C.: Climacteric continuous bleeding. Her menstruation has been irregular and liable to be prolonged for the last several months. This photograph shows the uterine cavity just before bleeding begins. The endometrium, which is thickened and undulated with many deep indentations of the glandular opening, is hardly collapsed

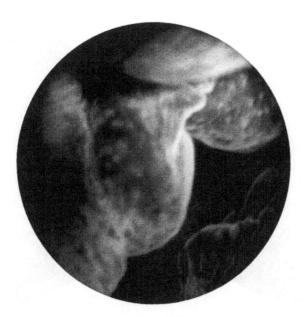

Fig. 98. Simple hyperplasia of the endometrium. Age 44. C.C.: Irregular menstruation. Patient had complained of recent irregular and prolonged menstruation. This photograph shows the uterine cavity just after bleeding began. Although the bleeding has begun, almost all the thickened endometrium is retained without sloughing, showing slight engorgement

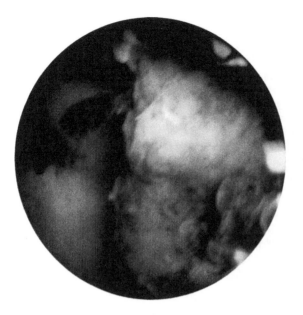 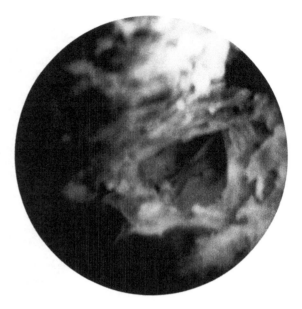

Fig. 99. Simple hyperplasia of the endometrium. Age 53. C.C.: Irregular bleeding, continuing for 10 days. Nearly all the endometrium is shed, leaving in part the thick polypous endometrium with ragged unrepaired surface

Fig. 100. Simple hyperplasia of the endometrium. Age 46. C.C.: Stubborn bleeding for a long time. Bleeding has continued for more than 45 days. The uterine cavity is full of necrotic fragments of the sloughed endometrium, but the partly stripped endometrium remains in the *upper right* of the photograph

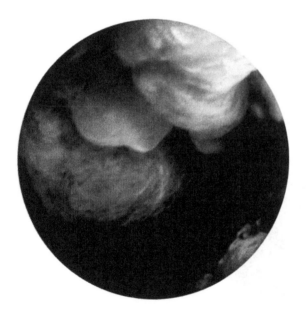 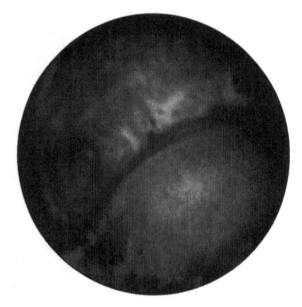

Fig. 101. Simple hyperplasia of the endometrium. Age 46. C.C.: Continual bleeding for a long time. Bleeding has lasted intermittently for 25 days. Nearly all the endometrium is sloughed, leaving part of the moundlike vegetating endometrium. This remaining endometrium, which has begun to remodel, resembles focal hyperplasia so that it is indiscernible without knowledge of the natural course of bleeding

Fig. 102. Focal hyperplasia of the endometrium. Age 56. C.C.: Increased whitish discharge. Arcuate eminence of the endometrium surrounded by atrophic endometrium is visible on the posterior wall of the uterus. Bleeding is not discernible

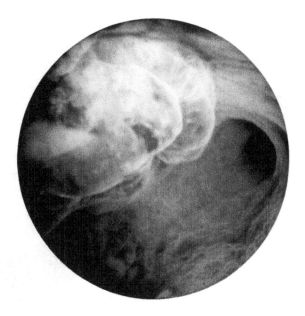

Fig. 103. Focal hyperplasia of the endometrium. Age 30. C.C.: Prolonged menstruation. Photograph taken at 9 days of the cycle. A solitary, polypous projection near the left tubal ostium is vivid in color and provides a feature of the endometrium in the proliferative phase

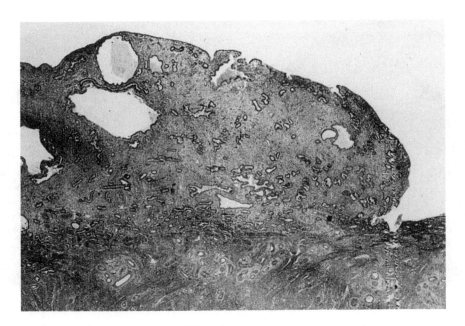

Fig. 104. Histology of focal hyperplasia of the endometrium. Age 60. Focal prominence of the endometrium with cystic hyperplasia adjoins the senile atrophic endometrium

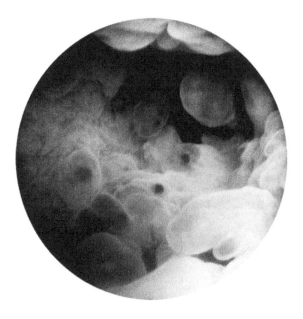
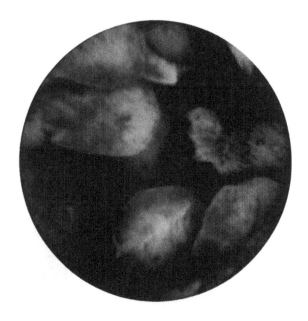

Fig. 105. Polypous hyperplasia of the endometrium. Age 30. C.C.: Midcycle spotting. Each projection of the polypous hyperplasia provides the feature of simple hyperplasia. Small blood spots appear on the tip of a few projections

Fig. 106. Polypous hyperplasia of the endometrium. Age 31. C.C.: Wish for childbearing and prolonged menstruation. Polypous endometrial projections with capillary engorgement fill the uterine cavity

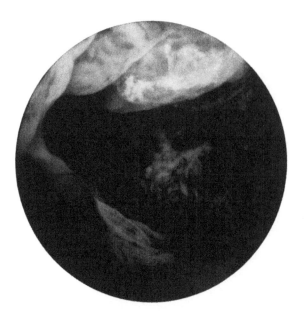
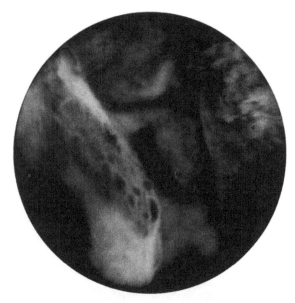

Fig. 107. Polypous hyperplasia of the endometrium. Age 42. C.C.: Intermittent slight bleeding. The patient has complained of slight bleeding followed by menorrhagia for the past 3 weeks. Some of the projections provide an atypical vascular network on the surface. A biopsied specimen showed atypical hyperplasia

Fig. 108. Polypous hyperplasia of the endometrium. Age 50. C.C.: Postmenopausal spotting. Her menopause occurred at age 48. Polypous projections are engorged; some of them have sporadic blood spots or atypical vessels

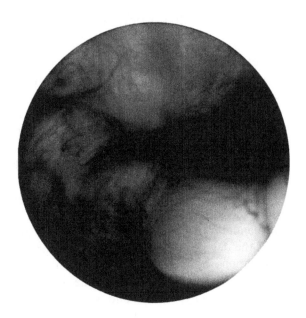

Fig. 109. Cystic hyperplasia of the endometrium. Age 60. C.C.: Postmenopausal spotting. Her menopause occurred at age 51. The endometrium itself is not hyperplastic, but the fornicate cystic gland, which appears translucent and *whitish* in color, bulges into the uterine cavity

7.2.3.2 High-Risk Endometrial Hyperplasia

High-risk hyperplasia is thought of as a premalignant state of the endometrium, and is divided into two types, adenomatous hyperplasia and atypical hyperplasia. This category histologically includes a variety of architectural abnormalities and cytological atypisms in various combinations and varying degrees of severity (Lawrence and Scully 1989). Although by using hysteroscopy it is rather difficult to differentiate these lesions, it is useful to perform target biopsy for the suspicious lesions selected by hysteroscopy. It seems that adenomatous hyperplasia has the characteristic that its cytology shows distinct atypism but it is poor in a particular view of hysteroscopy. In most cases of adenomatous hyperplasia, the endometrium is focally thickened. The lesion, which has an uneven surface because of crater formation of the glandular opening, is *yellow-red* in color and has few atypical vessels.

As the degree of gland atypism increases, atypical vessels are prominent, indentations of the gland opening faint, and projections polypous. As a matter of fact, in some instances, the hysteroscopic differentiation between severe atypical hyperplasia and well-differentiated adenocarcinoma is often difficult. Final diagnosis must await histopathological confirmation by target biopsy.

In some instances, women who have been diagnosed as high-risk endometrial hyperplasia by hysteroscopy and subsequent histology are likely to progress to endometrial carcinoma. In reproductive-age women, an attempt to follow up hysteroscopy should be made to judge whether a better or worse transition of the disease occurred following conservative medical and surgical treatment. A case with better effects and poorer outcomes is shown in Figs. 110–114a–d.

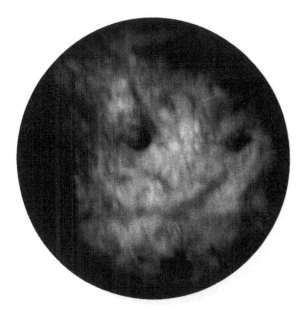

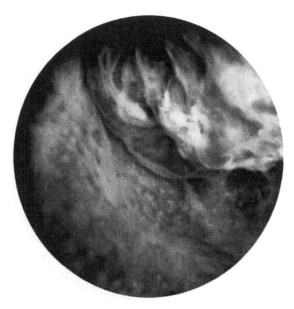

Fig. 110. Adenomatous hyperplasia of the endometrium. Age 48. C.C.: Abnormal bleeding. This picture was taken on day 16 of the cycle. The endometrium is almost shed, partly leaving the lower layer. The vascular pattern is not very marked, but dilated glandular openings are characteristic

Fig. 111. Partial adenomatous hyperplasia of the endometrium. Age 48. C.C.: Postmenstrual spotting. The patient has complained of intermittent spotting following her regular period. At the left cornu, a polypous projection with wrinkled surface is hanging. Glandular opening is hidden behind the wrinkles

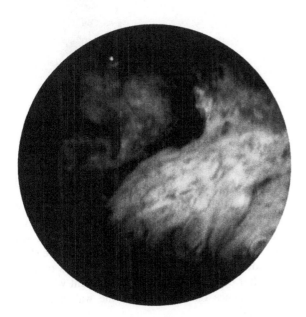

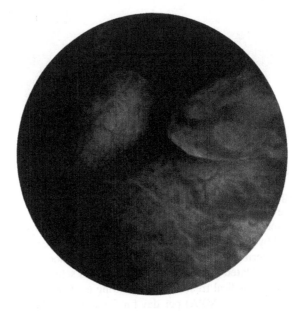

Fig. 112. Adenomatous hyperplasia of the endometrium. Age 48. C.C. Irregular bleeding. The patient has complained of continual spotting for several months. Hysteroscopy was done on day 142 after the onset of the bleeding. The endometrium is irregularly sloughed, and the rest shows focal hyperplasia of the endometrium with dilated glandular openings

Fig. 113. Atypical hyperplasia of the endometrium. Age 60. C.C.: Postmenopausal spotting. Her menopause occurred 8 years ago. Two lumps of focal hyperplasia of the endometrium show atypical blood vessels on the surface

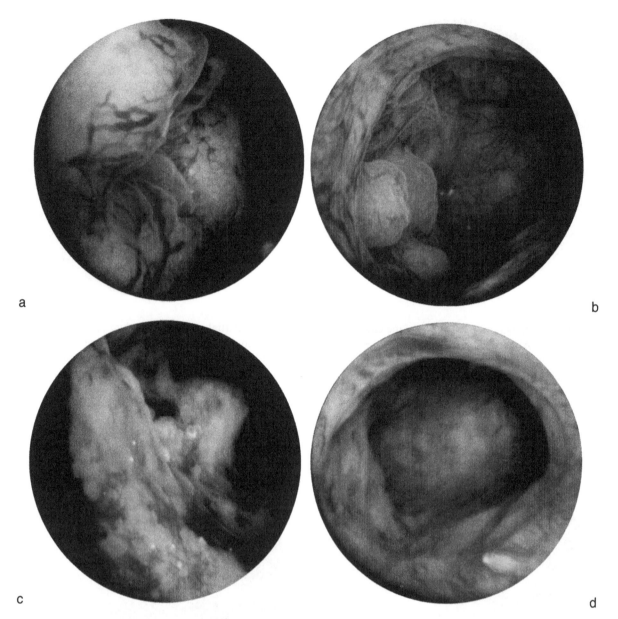

a

b

c

d

Fig. 114a–d. Atypical hyperplasia of the endometrium. Age 64. C.C.: Postmenopausal bleeding. The patient has complained of slight bleeding for the past 5 days. **a** Knobby prominence developed on the right uterine wall is characterized by the appearance of atypical blood vessels and no dilated glandular opening. She was scheduled to undergo medical treatment with 800 mg medroxyprogesterone acetate (MPA) per day for 3 months. **b** She was treated by medication with 800 mg MPA per day for 40 days. The size of the prominence and atypism of the vessels decreased fairly well. **c** She was medicated with 800 mg MPA per day for 85 days. The prominence shows much more shrinkage. **d** This photograph was taken on day 30 after completion of 90-day treatment with MPA. The prominence on the right uterine wall has almost disappeared

7.2.4 Endometrial Carcinoma

Most endometrial carcinomas are seen during both premenopausal and postmenopausal ages. Abnormal bleeding is the only symptom in about 90% of women with endometrial carcinoma. If speculum examination has led to the assessment that the bleeding in postmenopausal women is from the cervical canal, hysteroscopy should routinely be carried out. Apart from traditional fractional curettage and endometrial cytology, we are sure that hysteroscopy is an extremely reliable method for diagnosis of endometrial carcinoma, because often it exophytically grows into the uterine cavity and presents a characteristic appearance. Hysteroscopic diagnosis of endometrial carcinoma is made by means of macroscopic vision, for example, localization, extent, unevenness, color, and vascularity of irregular vegetation. On the basis of thorough knowledge of architectural features near the surface area of endometrial carcinoma, sufficient hysteroscopy enables us to presume histopatholgy of the disease.

As endometrial carcinoma often occurs in elderly women and is liable to be accompanied by bleeding and infection, attention should be directed to the following. (1) Hysteroscopy is the first procedure to be done before smear and tissue sampling, which may substantially distort the original appearance of the lesion. If these manipulations have been done already, a 7- to 10-day interval should precede hysteroscopy. (2) Cervical dilatation, if needed, is carefully done to prevent laceration. (3) Blood, pus, and debris are thoroughly removed by using rinsing fluid. (4) The pressure of endocavity irrigation is kept moderate to avoid peritoneal spillage of tumor cells in rinsing fluid through the tubes. (5) Endoscopy begins in the cervical canal with possible invasion of endometrial carcinoma before cervical dilatation. (6) Biopsy must be done on live lesions without necrosis.

Endometrial carcinoma is divided into four patterns according to the view of the tumor by means of panoramic hysteroscopy using a fluid distending medium; polypoid, nodular, papillomatous, and diffuse. More detailed examination enables us to predict architectural features of the lesion: tubular, adenomatous, and papillary adenocarcinoma. The majority of endometrial carcinomas are localized as adenocarcinomas, drawing a distinct line between the tumor and the surrounding atrophic endometrium. As carcinoma progresses, the surface becomes necrotized and ulcerated.

7.2.4.1 Polypoid Carcinoma

Histologically well-differentiated (e.g., tubular or adenomatous) adenocarcinoma produces a polypoid outgrowth with thin pedicles. The surface with a few atypical vessels is somewhat uneven, and the glandular opening is not prominent (Figs. 115–118). It appears *grayish-white* in color. The surface unevenness and atypical vascularity are more striking in adenomatous adenocarcinoma than in the tubular type (see Figs. 119, 120). Ulceration is rare.

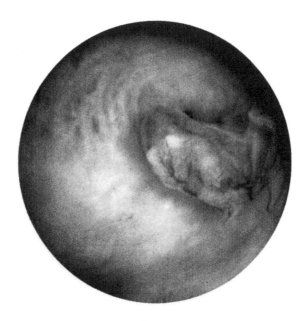

Fig. 115. Polypoid carcinoma of the endometrium. Age 66. Near the left tubal ostium solitary, a tiny polypoid carcinoma is growing. The surface, with atypical vessels that are not prominent, is flattened. Biopsy showed tubular adenocarcinoma, but no more cancer tissue in the hysterectomized specimen could be found

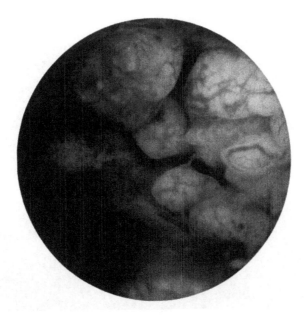

Fig. 116. Polypoid carcinoma of the endometrium. Age 38. The patient has wished for childbearing and had been diagnosed as polycystic ovary syndrome. Multiple polypoid projections show atypical vessels on the surface. As this finding tends to be confused with polypous hyperplasia of the endometrium, the final diagnosis depended on histopathological confirmation. Histology of this case showed tubular adenocarcinoma of the endometrium.

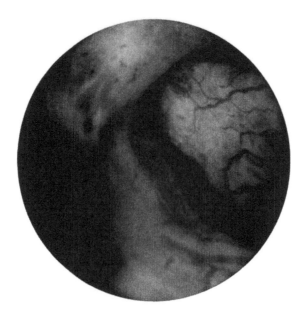

Fig. 117. Polypoid carcinoma of the endometrium. Age 58. Polypoid projection appears just in the inner part of the intact internal os. The surface of the tumor, which is characterized by atypical vessels and dilated glandular openings, is quite wavy. Histology showed adenomatous adenocarcinoma of the endometrium

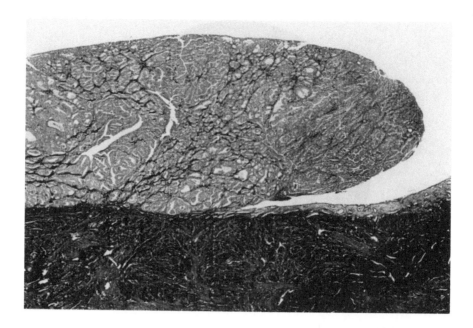

Fig. 118. Histology of adenomatous adenocarcinoma of the endometrium with polypoid growth. Age 46. Adenomatous carcinoma of the endometrium contrasts sharply with the surrounding atrophic endometrium

7.2.4.2 Nodular Carcinoma

Adenomatous adenocarcinoma often presents nodular patterns, correlated with the cerebroid type of carcinoma of Barbot (1989) (Figs. 119, 120). Atypical vascularity is so remarkable that it may often present varicosities that are heaped up tortuously from the surface (Figs. 121, 122). The surface of tubular adenocarcinoma with nodular growth is flattened, while adenomatous adenocarcinoma is rather ragged because of swelling of the glandular opening (Figs. 123–128). Although ulceration and infection are rare in the early stage, the frequency tends to increase as the stage advances (Fig. 126). It is important to differentiate this from submucosal leiomyoma displaying similar outgrowth (see Figs. 194–196, later in this chapter).

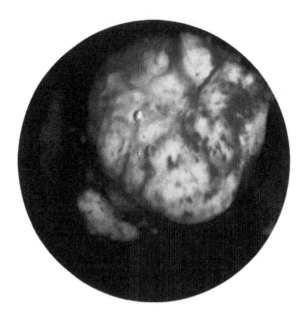

Fig. 119. Nodular carcinoma of the endometrium. Age 48. Two nodules protrude from the anterior wall of the uterus. The surface is rather ragged and characterized by swollen, *whitish* glandular openings

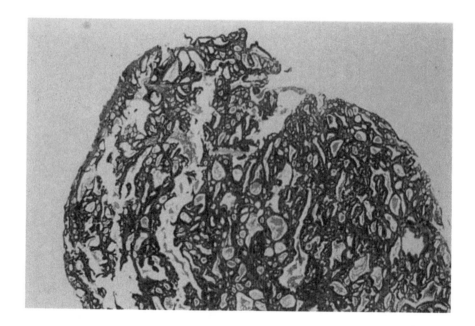

Fig. 120. Histology of adenomatous adenocarcinoma of the endometrium with nodular growth. Age 59. Glands of adenocarcinoma in various sizes account for the greater part of the tumor

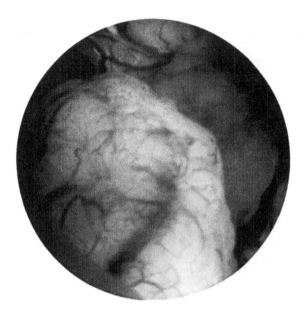

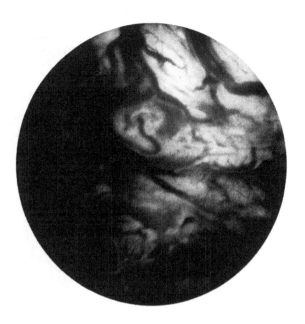

Fig. 121. Nodular carcinoma of the endometrium. Age 57. The surface of each nodule is not so ragged, and vascular atypism is not remarkable

Fig. 122. Nodular carcinoma of the endometrium. Age 51. This is one of the most characteristic features of nodular carcinoma of the endometrium: atypical vessels wind in a zigzag pattern on the suface of the tumor

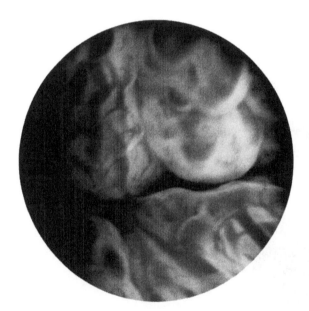

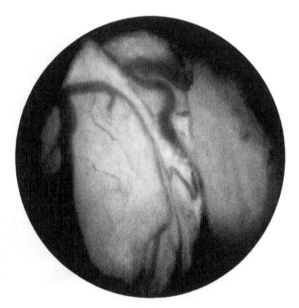

Fig. 123. Nodular carcinoma of the endometrium. Age 53. Sometimes atypical vessels may creep close together in a heap. In such a case, the glandular opening is often indistinct

Fig. 124. Nodular carcinoma of the endometrium. Age 52. Another hysteroscopic feature of nodular carcinoma is unevenness of the surface. The surface in this case is fairly flattened exept for a tiny part of the right side with a ragged surface. Histologically, the flat portion frequently indicates tubular adenocarcinoma and the ragged portion often shows adenomatous adenocarcinoma

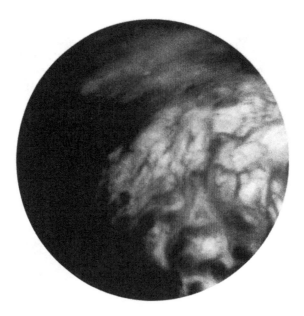

Fig. 125. Nodular carcinoma of the endometrium. Age 68. Almost all the surface of the tumor presents granular unevenness because of a swelling of glandular openings surrounded by atypical vessels. Histology showed adenomatous adenocarcinoma

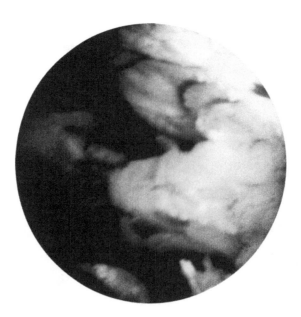

Fig. 126. Nodular carcinoma of the endometrium. Age 59. Only a few nodular carcinomas of the endometrium display focal necrosis. With increasing necrosis of the tumor, the characteristic appearance of nodular carcinoma is gradually diminished

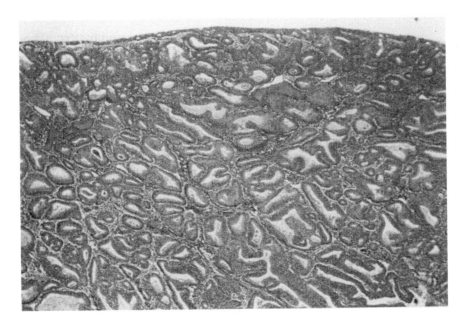

Fig. 127. Histology of tubular adenocarcinoma of the endometrium with nodular growth. Age 46. The free surface of the tumor is flattened and subepithelial vessels are not conspicuous

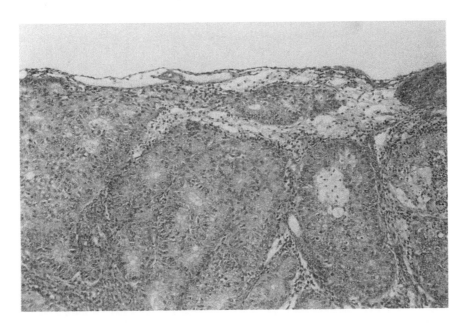

Fig. 128. Histopathology of adenomatous adenocarcinoma of the endometrium with nodular growth. Age 59. The free surface of the tumor is quite irregular. Subepithelial veins, although shriveled by formalin fixation, are characteristic

7.2.4.3 Papillomatous Carcinoma

Papillomatous carcinoma is the most common pattern of endometrial carcinoma, found in half or more of patients when examination is performed by using panoramic hysteroscopy with a fluid distending medium, unlike contact or CO_2 hysteroscopy. The tumor apparently looks like a nodular cluster (Figs. 129–131), but further detailed examination discloses that the surface is covered with numerous tentacle-like projections of cancerous structures quivering in the rinsing fluid (Figs. 132–136). These tentacles, some long and others short, gather and form a dendritic mass. Each tentacle with a tint of *light pink* shows the very image of the properties of cancerous tissue proliferating around the stroma involved with dilated blood vessels during hysteroscopy. Short tentacles resemble clusters of grapes (Figs. 137, 138), and long ones interlocking with each other look like balls of yarn. Thus, recognition of papillomatous carcinoma by hysteroscopy is pathognomonic and accurate.

Most endometrial carcinomas are a blend of these patterns in the same instance (Figs. 139–141). The most common pattern is mostly papillomatous and partly nodular. Histopathological pictures near the free surface of a papillomatous carcinoma of the endometrium are shown in Figs. 142–146. Papillomatous carcinoma of the endometrium is also liable to deteriorate into necrosis and infection, resulting in focal ulceration, which often leads to confusing the exact diagnosis by using hysteroscopy (Figs. 147, 148).

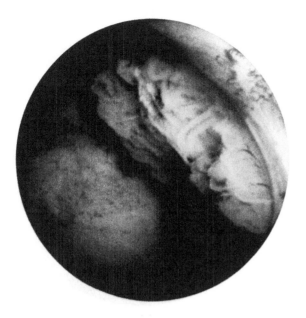
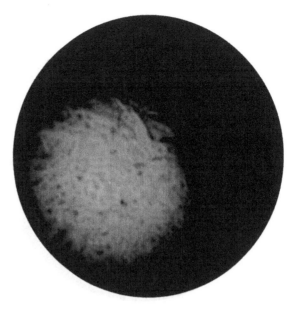

Fig. 129. Early papillomatous carcinoma of the endometrium. Age 57. At the left cornu, a nodule of papillomatous carcinoma appears. The tiny tumor consists of intertwined tentacle-like projections

Fig. 130. Early papillomatous carcinoma of the endometrium. Age 70. Near the left tubal ostium, there is a ball-like projection, the surface of which is overlaid with many short processes

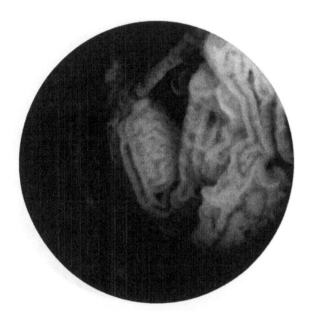
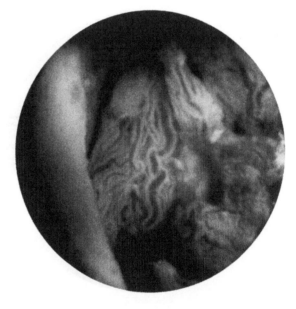

Fig. 131. Papillomatous carcinoma of the endometrium. Age 56. Although the tumor reveals ball-like growth as a whole, some long tentacle-like projections away from the surface are quivering in the rinsing fluid

Fig. 132. Papillomatous carcinoma of the endometrium. Age 53. The greater part of the tentacle-like projections on the surface of the tumor swing in the fluid

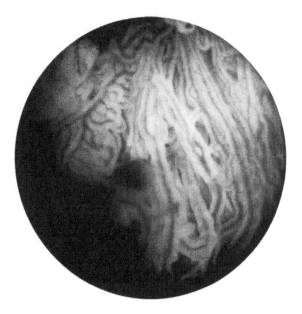

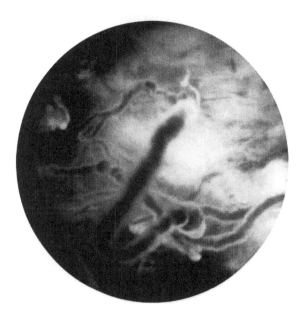

Fig. 133. Papillomatous carcinoma of the endometrium. Age 54. Very long tentacle-like projections freely sway in the fluid. Each projection, which consists of a *pink* blood vessel surrounded by cancer structure, characteristically is identified histologically as papillary adenocarcinoma

Fig. 134. Papillomatous carcinoma of the endometrium. Age 53. Free tentacles may appear quivering in the rinsing fluid

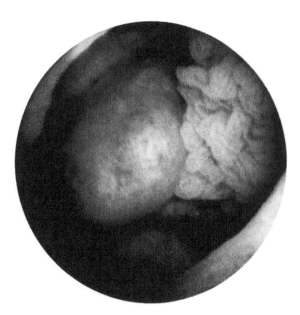

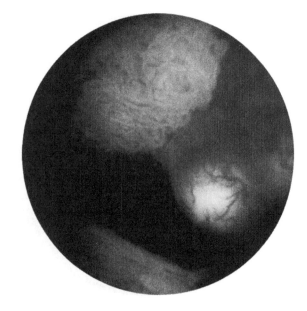

Fig. 135. Papillomatous carcinoma and benign polyp of the endometrium. Age 52. Typical endometrial polyp coexists with papillomatous endometrial carcinoma. Bleeding was caused by collapsed papillary tentacles of carcinoma

Fig. 136. Papillomatous carcinoma of the endometrium and submucosal fibroid. Age 49. Menorrhagia may result from endometrial carcinoma not but coexistent submucosal fibroid. This case showed negative intracavitary cytosmear and blind curettage. Behind a large submucosal fibroid, a small papillomatous carcinoma is hidden

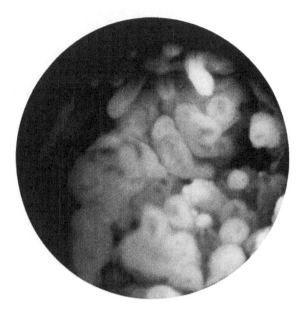 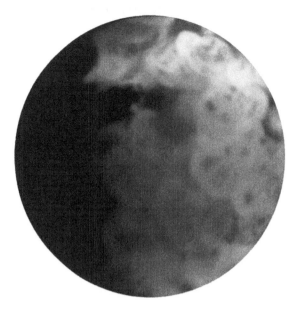

Fig. 137. Papillomatous carcinoma of the endometrium. Age 65. Tentacle-like projections are short, although the central blood vessels are hard to discern

Fig. 138. Papillomatous carcinoma of the endometrium. Age 46. Short globular processes with central vascular punctation grow in a cluster

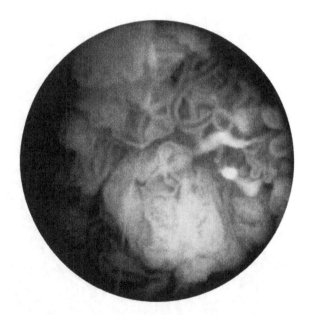 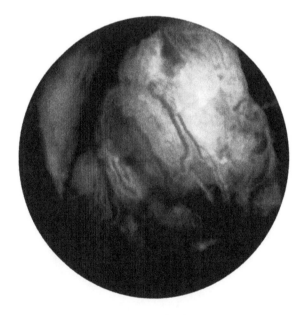

Fig. 139. Coexistence of nodular carcinoma of the endometrium with papillomatous carcinoma. Age 60. Cancer mass is a mix of nodular and papillomatous parts, half and half

Fig. 140. Coexistence of nodular carcinoma of the endometrium with papillomatous carcinoma. Age 53. Nodular carcinoma of the endometrium is partly papillomatous

Fig. 141. Nodular carcinoma of the endometrium shows partial papillary growth. Age 54

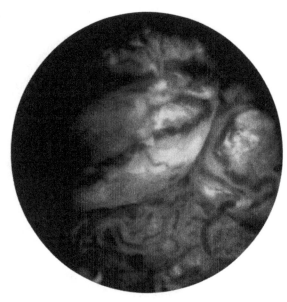

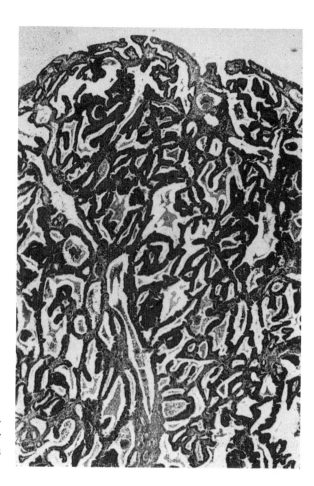

Fig. 142. Longitudinal section of papillary adenocarcinoma of the endometrium. Age 60. Short papillary projections stick out from the free surface of papillomatous carcinoma of the endometrium with nodular growth

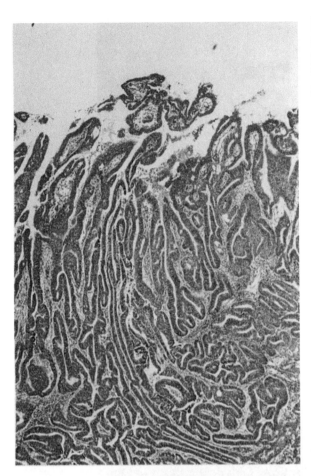

Fig. 143. Longitudinal section of papillary adeno-carcinoma of the endometrium. Age 50. Many tentacle-like projections of carcinoma stick out into the free surface. As the relationship of glandular epithelium and the stroma is reversed, the glands surround the stroma

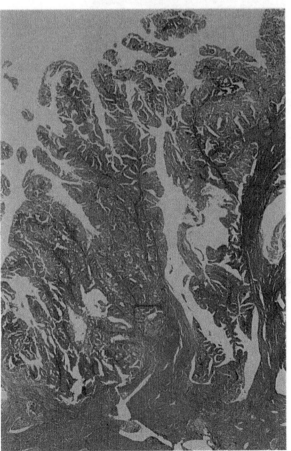

Fig. 144. Longitudinal section of papillary adeno-carcinoma of the endometrium. Age 63. Papillary adenocarcinoma vividly extends dendritically to the out-side. The trunks of the stroma are compact

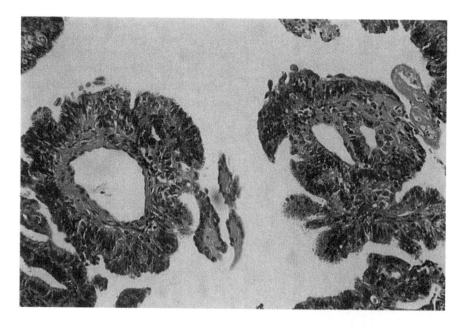

Fig. 145. Cross section of papillary adenocarcinoma of the endometrium. Age 51. Irregularly arranged cancer cells surround the stroma compressed by dilated vessels

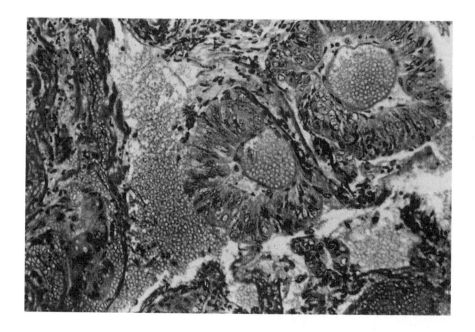

Fig. 146. Cross section of papillary adenocarcinoma of the endometrium. Age 68. Each tentacle consists of vivid cancer cells surrounding the stroma, extremely compressed by dilated veins filled with red blood cell thrombi

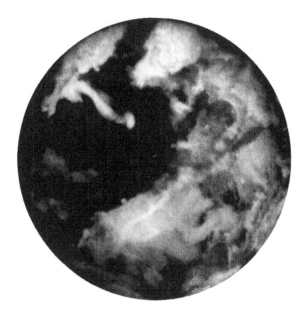

Fig. 147. Ulcerated papillomatous carcinoma of the endometrium complicated by pyometra. Age 61. Almost all the structure loses inherent features of papillomatous carcinoma, exept for the dilated vascular image, which is the only evidence of malignancy

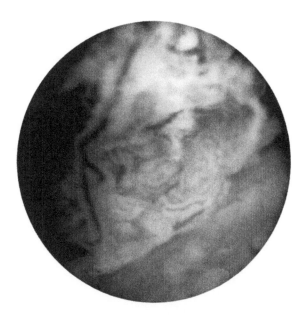

Fig. 148. Ulcerated papillomatous carcinoma of the endometrium. Age 63. Previous to the hysteroscopic examination, pus was washed out of the uterine cavity with rinsing saline. Hairy blood vessels appear among the frail structure of cancer

7.2.4.4 Diffuse Carcinoma

Diffuse carcinoma of the endometrium, although it occurs rather rarely, involves endophytically almost the entire uterine lining (Fig. 149). The only hysteroscopic finding is the formation of ulcers in which there are few features peculiar to endometrial carcinoma besides striking atypical vascularity. Diffuse carcinoma is often poorly differentiated. It may be difficult to discriminate this finding from that of the lesion which has been thoroughly curetted for histological diagnosis before hysteroscopic examination (Fig. 150). On the other hand, circumscribed endometrial carcinoma may also display diffuse outgrowth when the extent and infection of the disease result in ulceration. Metastatic endometrial carcinoma often may show duffuse development (Fig. 151).

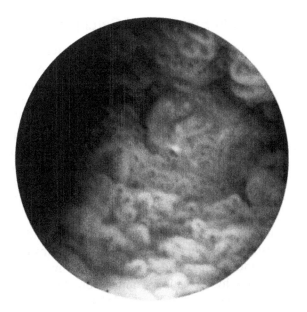

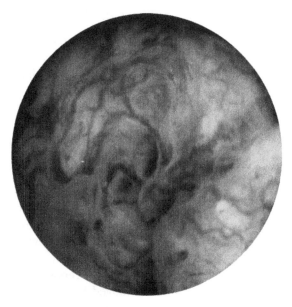

Fig. 149. Diffuse endometrial carcinoma. Age 54. This is a rare case with diffuse papillomatous carcinoma of the endometrium that has spread throughout the uterine lining

Fig. 150. Endometrial carcinoma curetted before hysteroscopy. Age 64. The picture seems to show diffuse carcinoma of the endometrium at first sight, but actually the patient was thoroughly curetted 7 days previously and the original feature was almost lost

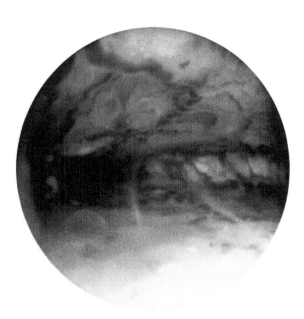

Fig. 151. Metastatic endometrial carcinoma. Age 38. This patient underwent an operation for gastric carcinoma 2 years previously and has complained of slight genital bleeding for about a week. The lining mucosa is thoroughly thin and ragged, but provides atypical vessels

7.2.4.5 Cervical Involvement in Endometrial Carcinoma

Another advantage of hysteroscopy is detection of cervical extension of endometrial carcinoma (Figs. 152–154). As described previously, it is absolutely essential that hysteroscopy for examining the cervical canal should be performed before cervical dilatation to avoid tissue distortion. The internal os of the normal uterus is clearly demarcated and shows a smooth circular opening. There are two aspects of cervical spread of endometrial carcinoma, cervical glandular involvement (stage IIA) and cervical stromal invasion (stage IIB). The cervical effect is usually accompanied by glandular involvement detectable by using endoscopy (Figs. 155–157). Cervical invasive carcinoma looks *grayish-yellow* and irregular, because it is usually modified by ulceration and necrosis by infection and makes the circular internal os distorted. In instances in which only the stromal invasion is lacking in glandular involvement, however, diagnosis is unreliable by means of hysteroscopy (Fig. 158), requiring the help of CT and MRI. Because the depth of myometrial invasion remains unknown by using hysteroscopic examination, it should be judged by endoscopic ultrasonography (US), CT, and MRI at the present time.

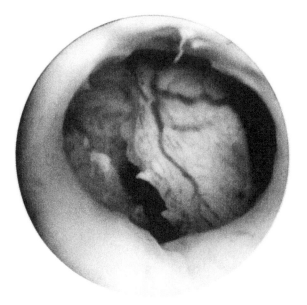

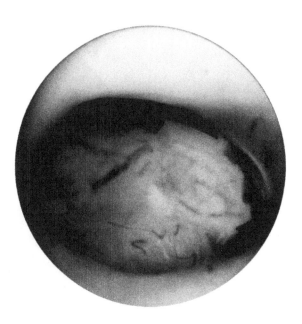

Fig. 152. Endometrial carcinoma without cervical invasion. Age 63. The cervical internal os is saved from cancer involvement and sustains the smooth, round circle of the internal os

Fig. 153. Endometrial carcinoma without cervical invasion. Age 66. The tip of polypoid carcinoma of the endometrium is ulcerated and extends to the internal os of the cervix, which is free from invasion of carcinoma

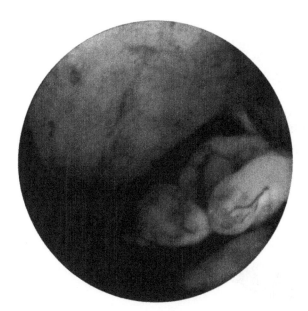

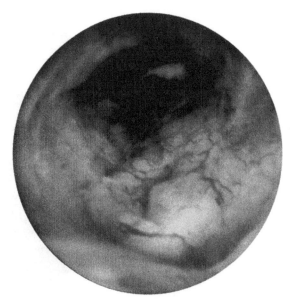

Fig. 154. Endometrial carcinoma without cervical invasion. Age 72. Polypoid carcinoma of the endometrium lies beyond the internal os of the cervix without cancer involvement. This actually is in stage I of endometrial carcinoma, but there is some fear that blind biopsy of the cervix may lead to misdiagnosis of stage I carcinoma as stage 11 carcinoma

Fig. 155. Nodular carcinoma of the endometrium with cervical involvement. Age 53. Cancer involvement to the cervix can be seen at 3 to 7 o'clock

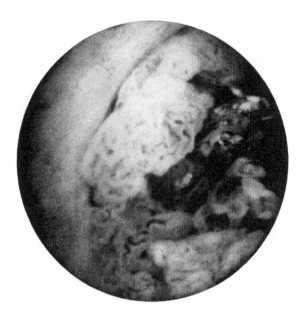

Fig. 156. Papillomatous carcinoma with cervical involvement. Age 60. Cancer involvement to the cervix is recognized at 6 to 7 o'clock

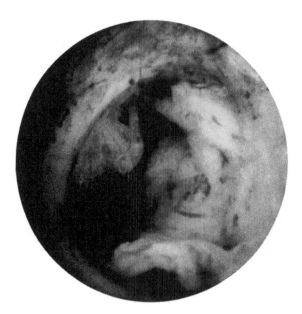

Fig. 157. Nodular carcinoma with cervical invasion. Age 73. The left half of the internal os is distorted because of cancer invasion

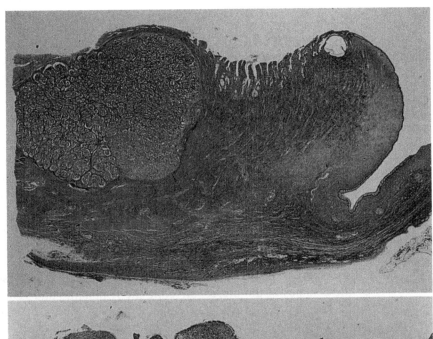

a

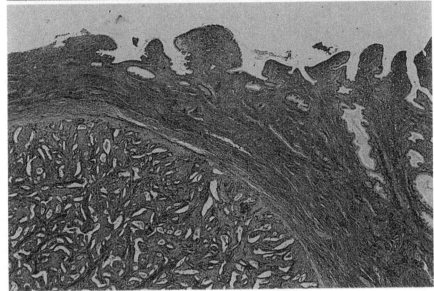

b

Fig. 158a,b. Histopathology of cervical stromal invasion lacking in glandular involvement in a case of endometrial carcinoma. Age 64. **a** Although carcinoma invades the stroma beneath the cervical isthmus, the lining endocervix is intact. In such a case, cervical invasion of endometrial carcinoma, if any, cannot be detected by hysteroscopy. **b** Detail of cervical stromal invasion harbored with the intact endocervix

7.2.5 Nonepithelial Neoplasia of the Endometrium

It is uncommon to encounter a patient with a nonepithelial neoplasia of the endometrium on hysteroscopic examination. This affects perimenopausal or postmenopausal women predominantly, leading to abnormal uterine bleeding. Judging from our little experience, it is impossible to use hysteroscopy to discern each origin of nonepithelial neoplasia; myometrial, stromal, and mixed patterns, including both epithelial and mesodermal elements. However, it is possible with much experience that hysteroscopy can be used to discriminate between pure endometrial carcinoma and other mesodermal malignancy. It grows exophytically in a polypoid or nodular fashion, occasionally to fill the uterine cavity. The tumor is often soft and fragile. The surface of the tumor is uneven, opaque, and dull *grayish-yellow* in color, lacking in markedly atypical vessels. Endometrial stromal neoplasia can be classified into two main types: the first is borderline malignancy (that is, stromal endometriosis) (Fig. 159), and the second undoubtedly is sarcomatous (that is, stromal sarcoma) (Figs. 160a–d). Both stromal endometriosis and stromal sarcoma are infiltrative and spread beyond the confines of the uterus, affecting the lymphatics and veins, although the latter is more aggressive. Another unique anaplastic neoplasia of the endometrium is the tumor having malignancy of both epithelial and nonepthelial elements.

In addition to a carcinoma of mesodermal type, the most common carcinomas include such as endometriod, clear cell, or squamous cell carcinoma. The first is mixed with malignancy of the stroma, that is, stromal sarcoma, composed of malignant elements of tissue native to the uterus (carcinosarcoma of the endometrium) (Figs. 161–164). The second is mixed with heterologous sarcoma of the uterus, that is, it contains neoplastic elements of tissue not native to the uterus, namely rhabdomyosarcomatous, chondrosarcomatous, and osteosarcomatous elements (heterologous mixed mesodermal tumor of the endometrium) (Fig. 165a–c). In any case, hysteroscopy is merely a means to discriminate nonepithelial malignancy of the endometrium from pure endometrial carcinoma. Precise diagnosis must await histopathological confirmation, performing a biopsy and moreover serial sections of hysterectomized specimens to exclude a diagnosis of pure adenocarcinoma of the endometrium.

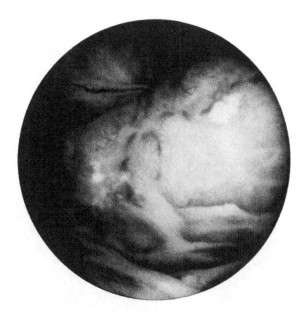

Fig. 159. Stromal endometriosis. Age 53. C.C.: Postmenopausal bleeding. A soft polypoid tumor with fairly sessile peduncle bulges into the uterine cavity. The surface is ragged and dull, *reddish-yellow* in color, unlike a benign endometrial polyp. Histology showed endolymphatic stromatosis

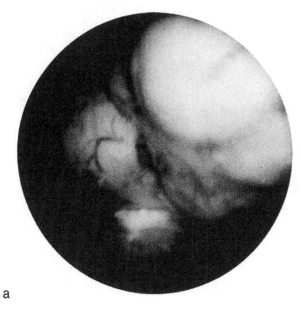

Fig. 160a–d. Stromal sarcoma. Age 41. C.C.: Irregular menstruation. **a** The uterine cavity is full of lumpy nodules, the surface of which looks dull *white* in color because of poor vascularization. **b** Gross appearance of stromal sarcoma in hysterectomized specimen. The tumor consists of an aggregate of nodules that vary in size. **c** Histopathology of stromal sarcoma. The tumor permeates the lymph vessels in a linguiform fashion. **d** Details of stromal sarcoma. The tumor is composed of sheets of anaplastic stromal cells, partially with mitotic activity

a

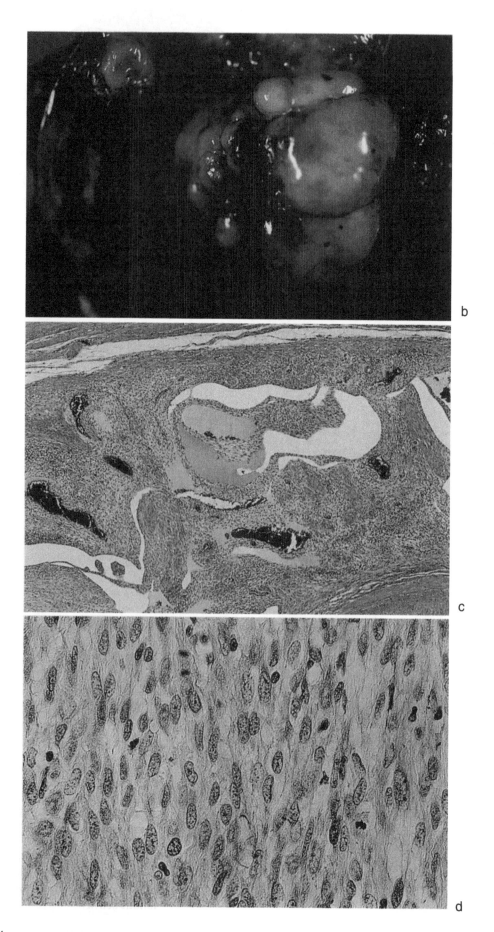

b

c

d

Fig. 160. Continued.

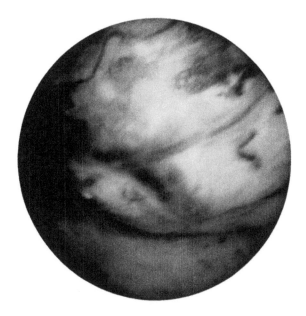

Fig. 161. Carcinosarcoma of the endometrium. Age 79. C.C.: Postmenopausal bleeding. Nodular mass protrudes into the uterine cavity. Dilated vessels are rather deeper than those of nodular carcinoma

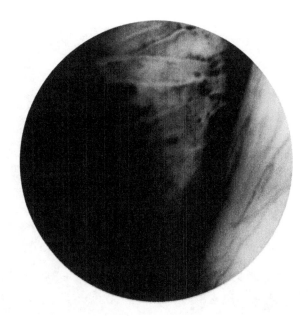

Fig. 162. Carcinosarcoma of the endometrium. Age 70. Hysteroscopy demonstrates the irregular surface with punctate small blood spots. Atypical vessels are not remarkable

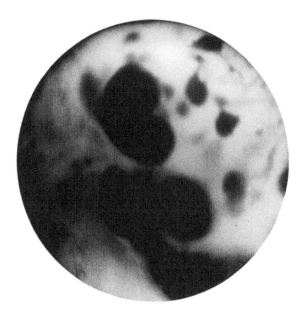

Fig. 163. Carcinosarcoma of the endometrium. Age 59. C.C.: Copious bleeding after menopause. Somewhat swollen blood spots of various sizes appear on the surface with *whitish* tint

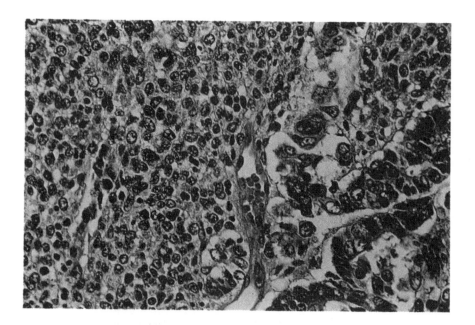

Fig. 164. Histopathology of carcinosarcoma of the endometrium. Endometrioid carcinoma of the endometrium (*right half*) borders on a highly cellular stroma with mitotic figures (*left half*)

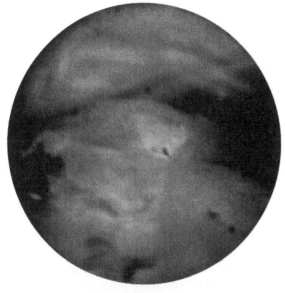

a

Fig. 165a–c. Mixed mesodermal tumor of the endometrium. Age 81. C.C.: Postmenopausal spotting. **a** Necrotic mass with the uneven and poorly vascularized surface is located on the posterior wall of the uterus. Heterologous malignancy mixed with mesodermal tumor of the endometrium could not be identified until histopathology of hysterectomized specimen testified it. **b** Chondrosarcomatous element. A focus of chondrosarcoma is surrounded by stromal sarcoma. **c** Rhabdomyosarcomatous element. Phosphotungustic-hematoxylin stain

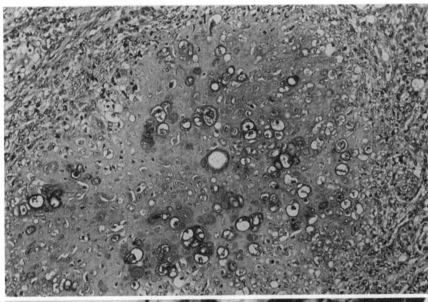

b

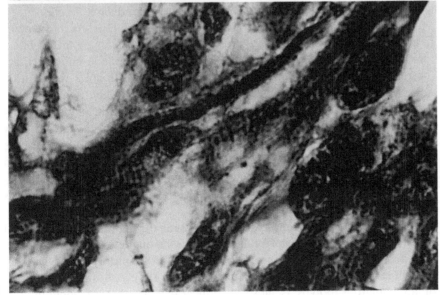

c

7.2.6 Endometrial Polyp

"Polyp" is usually defined as a new growth with a pedicle or a peduncle. Endometrial polyps are benign pedunculated growths bulging from the endometrial tissue alone. The peduncle is usually thin. The appearance is so close to that of submucosal myoma, polypoid endometrial carcinoma, and placental polyp that it is necessary to discriminate by using hysteroscopy cautiously. The lesions of endometrial polyps may be often asymptomatic; however, they occasionally cause abnormal uterine bleeding. Therefore, polyps may be found in the course of an infertility evaluation such as a hysterogram with filling defect or distorted contours. Although endometrial polyps occur in any age group, these in reproductive-age women are often functional and those in premenopausal to postmenopausal women are usually nonfunctional.

The functional polyp consists of a mucosa responsive to ovarian hormones, and their appearance is similar to that of the surrounding endometrium. It is generally small, and occurs anywhere on the uterine lining (Figs. 166, 167). Because its color and vasculature so closely resemble those of the surrounding endometrium, it may be mistaken for focal hyperplasia of the endometrium, which has a rather sessile base (see Figs. 102–104). A part of the polyp may participate in menstrual shedding, responding to progesterone.

The nonfunctional polyps grow in response to estrogen but not to progesterone. Peterson and Novak (1956) divided these polyps into three categories: retrogressive, typical, and adenomatous polyps.

Retrogressive polyps have a multilocular architecture similar to a cystic gland of Speert (1949), which is one of senile alteration. Speert described that these were a sort of retention cyst caused by occlusion of the glandular opening, containing mucus and debris. These cystic polyps are globular protrusions with a short pedicle, in striking contrast to the atrophic surrounding endometrium. They look *milky-white* in color and translucent (Figs. 168, 169). In the border of each loculus of the polyps, fine vasculature can be seen through the thin and friable wall. The wall seems to be easily broken even by a slight irritation, resulting in persistent postmenopausal bleeding (Figs. 170, 171).

Typical polyps have a structure histologically similar to cystic glandular hyperplasia of the endometrium of Schroeder (1934) (see Figs. 196, 197, later in this chapter). They mostly appear in the late reproductive to climacteric age, and range from tiny projections less than a few millimeters in diameter to large masses that occupy the entire uterine cavity. Although the architecture is similar to that of cystic glandular hyperplasia of the endometrium, these polyps hysteroscopically look *yellow-red* to *livid* in color with a little uneven surface, making a contrast with the adjacent endometrium harmonious with the menstrual cycle (Figs. 172–174). A pedicle of the polyp is usually thin, although it is occasionally sessile (Figs. 175–177). A typical polyp usually grows solitarily, but they may sometimes be multiple (Fig. 178). When the polyp grows quite near the tubal ostium, even if it is tiny, it may interfere with tubal patency (Figs. 179–181). A polyp does not always cause uterine bleeding. However, it may provoke persistent bleeding if ulceration and necrosis occur (Figs. 182–186).

Adenomatous polyps can be occasionally seen during the perimenopausal age. They are not as large in size, less than 1 cm in diameter, and have a short and wide-based pedicle. The appearance hysteroscopically is *red* with an uneven surface and poor vascularity (Figs. 187, 188). A hysteroscopic view of adenomatous polyps is close in appearance to that of adenomatous hyperplasia of the endometrium, while on the other hand it is also similar to polypous endometrial carcinoma. In particular, if it is very close to the latter, it is necessary to perform a detailed histological examination and a meticulous follow-up study using hysterocopy.

Endometrial polyps diagnosed by hysteroscopy are recovered en bloc under hysteroscopic guidance and subjected to a more accurate histological diagnosis. Second-look hysteroscopy is advisable to ensure that the uterus has been thoroughly emptied.

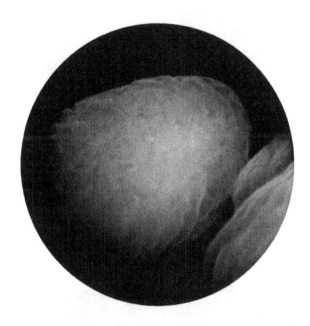

Fig. 166. Functional polyp of the endometrium in the midluteal phase. Age 39. C.C.: Premenstrual spotting. Hysteroscopy sights a tiny polyp with a wrinkled and tinted surface similar to the surrounding secretory endometrium (*lower right*)

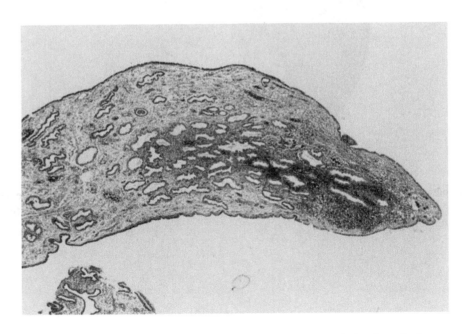

Fig. 167. Histopathology of functional polyp in the midluteal phase. Serrated glands and edematous stroma with bleeding reveal a secretory feature of the endometrium

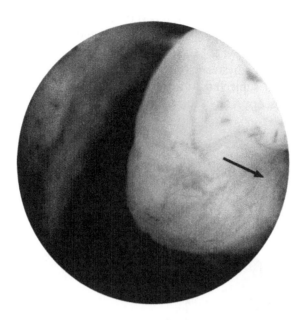

Fig. 168. Cystic polyp of the endometrium. Age 64. C.C.: Postmenopausal spotting. Pale polyp with the flattened surface is easily dented by blowing of rinsing fluid on hysteroscopy (*arrow*)

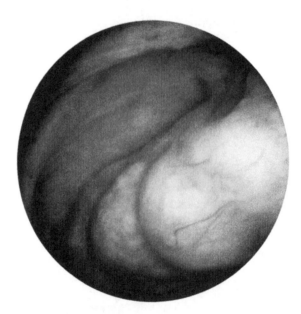

Fig. 169. Multiple cystic polyps of the endometrium. Age 67. C.C.: Postmenopausal bleeding. Three *whitish*, translucent polyps arranged side by side grow from the left wall of the uterus. The surface of the polyp in the foreground is dented by blowing of rinsing fluid

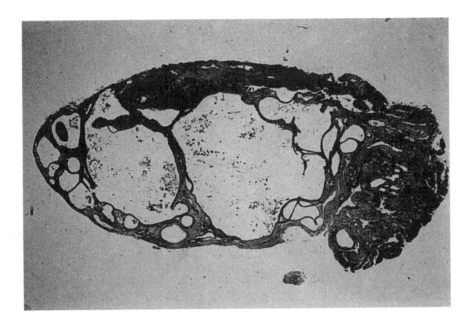

Fig. 170. Longitudinal section of cystic polyp of the endometrium. Many dilated glands forming multilocular cysts extremely oppress the surrounding stroma

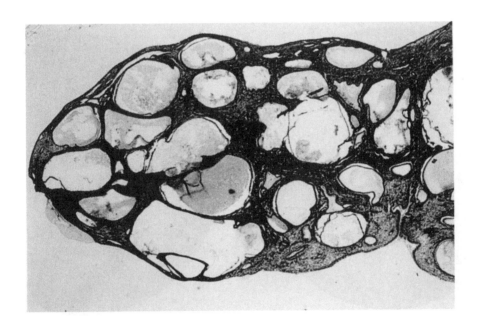

Fig. 171. Longitudinal section of cystic polyp of the endometrium. Mallory trichrome stain

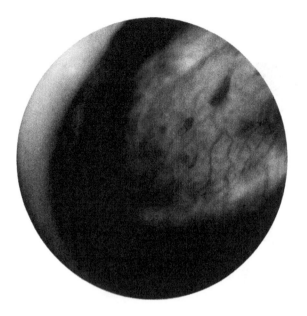

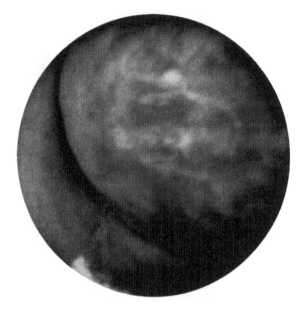

Fig. 172. Typical polyp of the endometrium. Age 53. C.C.: Postmenopausal spotting. The surface of typical polyp shows gentle undulation and has hairy vessels with blood spots in places

Fig. 173. Typical polyp of the endometrium. Age 37. C.C.: Prolonged menstruation and infertility. Ultrasonography (USG) and hysterosalpingography (HSG) suggested an intracavitary mass. The uterine cavity is almost full of congested typical polyp

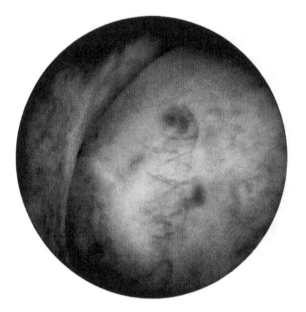

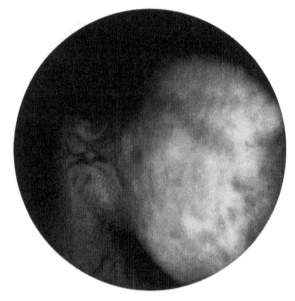

Fig. 174. Typical polyp of the endometrium. Age 49. C.C.: Postmenopausal bleeding. A large spherical polyp entirely fills the uterine cavity. Indentation and elasticity by pushing of the tip of hysteroscope suggests that this tumor is an endometrial polyp with soft and fragile properties. The surrounding endometrium is atrophic

Fig. 175. Pedicle of typical polyp of the endometrium. Age 52. C.C.: Postmenopausal bleeding. The pedicle of this spherical polyp is thin and surrounded by hairy blood vessels

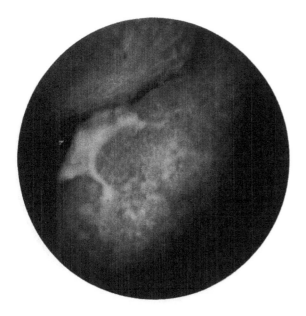

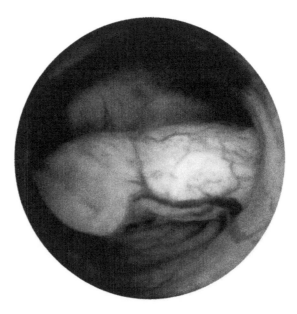

Fig. 176. Pedicle of typical polyp of the endometrium. Age 44. C.C.: Spotting. Polyp is long as a whole and the pedicle is also thin

Fig. 177. Pedicle of typical polyp of the endometrium. Age 45. C.C.: Spotting. Polyp shows uniform thickness from the tip to the root. Note subepithelial vessels, regularly arranged

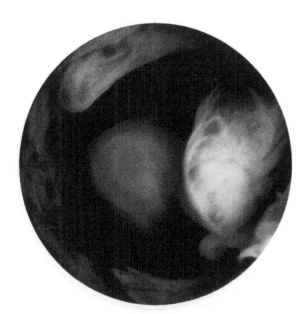

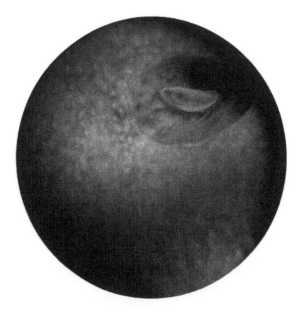

Fig. 178. Multiple typical polyp of the endometrium. Age 49. C.C.: Prolonged bleeding. Polyps of various sizes grow into the uterine cavity. It is difficult to discriminate a multiple typical polyp from polypoid hyperplasia of the endometrium by hysteroscopy

Fig. 179. Tiny polyp located near the tubal ostium. Age 30. C.C.: Wish for childbearing. A tiny polyp stands like a gatekeeper of the left tube. Hysterosalpingogram showed no image of the left tube

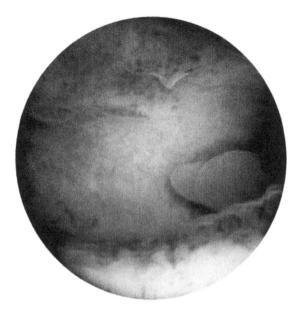

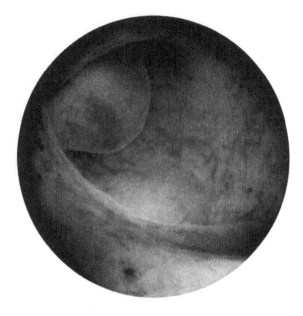

Fig. 180. Tiny polyps located near the left tubal ostium. Age 36. C.C.: Wish for childbearing. Polyp completely blocks the left tubal ostium. This case also had a similar polyp at another tubal ostium

Fig. 181. Typical polyp buried in the right tubal ostium. Age 35. C.C.: Wish for childbearing. A round small polyp is buried in the dilated right tubal ostium

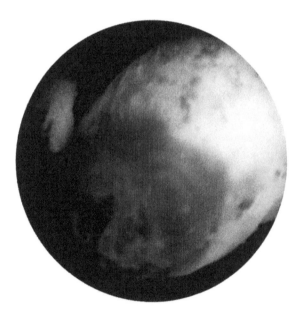

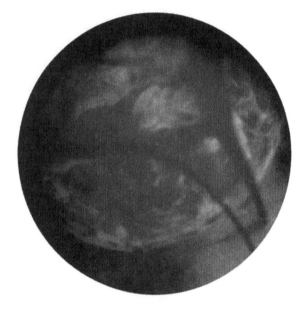

Fig. 182. Ulceration of typical polyp of the endometrium. Age 45. C.C.: Stubborn bleeding. The tip of this typical polyp is congested and partly broken off because of prolonged bleeding

Fig. 183. Typical polyp under profuse bleeding. Age 55. C.C.: Postmenopausal bleeding. The surface of the typical polyp is rough and engorged, showing lively bleeding

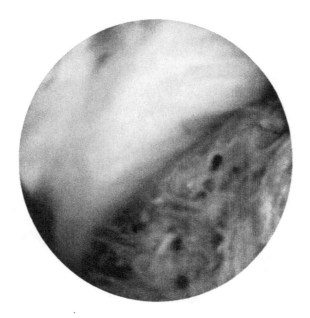

Fig. 184. Necrosed typical polyp. Age 58. C.C.: Increase in postmenopausal brown discharge. Tumor is rough, dull, and *brown*, in stark contrast to the surrounding atrophic endometrium

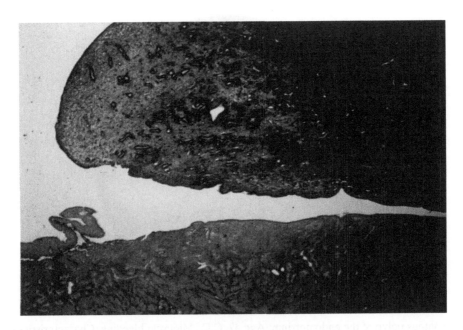

Fig. 185. Histopathology of typical polyp of the endometrium. The stroma is fibrous, and the glands resemble most closely the basal glands of the surrounding endometrium (*bottom*)

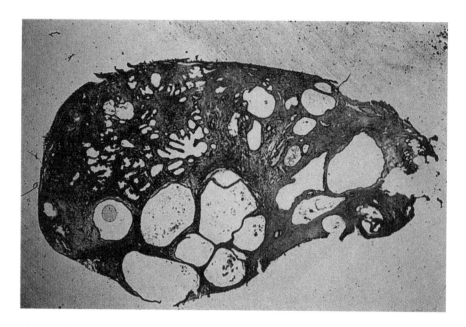

Fig. 186. Histopathology of typical polyp of the endometrium. Compact stroma and glands with variability in sizes look exactly like the 'Swiss cheese' pattern of endometrial hyperplasia of Schroeder

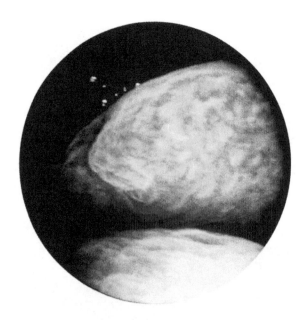

Fig. 187. Adenomatous polyp of the endometrium. Age 42. C.C.: Midcycle bleeding. Characteristics of adenomatous polyp are a fairly rough surface with dilated glandular openings that appear *white* in color

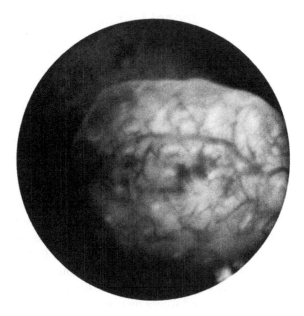

Fig. 188. Adenomatous polyp of the endometrium. Age 40. C.C.: Prolonged menstruation. In addition to the characteristics of adenomatous polyp, subepithelial blood vessels surrounding the glandular openings are peculiar

7.2.7 Submucosal Leiomyoma

Uterine leiomyomas are the most common tumors of the uterus, occurring in 25%–30% of reproductive-age women. Above all, submucosal leiomyomas, although not growing as rapidly in size, are often associated with infertility and persistent uterine bleeding. Common submucosal leiomyoma has been conventionally estimated by using imaging techniques such as hysterosalpingography (HSG), US, CT, and MRI. Hysteroscopic examination almost never misses submucosal leiomyoma as the hemispheric eminence to the globular mass on stalk bulging into the uterine cavity. These appear as round masses that bulge to varying extent toward the uterine cavity. When they bulge hemispherically toward the uterine cavity, the uterine cavity is deformed and the overlaying endometrium may occasionally present cyclic changes similar to those of the surrounding endometrium and sloughs during menstruation (Fig. 189–193). However, they ordinarily form hard pedunculated tumors, and sometimes may appear as livid, firm, polypoid masses in the vagina through the external cervical os. Thus, those leiomyomas are easily detected solely by using speculum examination.

The overlaying endometrium of pedunculated submucosal leiomyoma is ordinarily thin and lighter in color than the surrounding endometrium. A network of dilated vessels often displays regular arrangement, but occasionally it may be very scanty (Figs. 194–199). As leiomyoma grows with a peduncle, the overlaying endometrium becomes thin, ulcerated, hemorrhagic, and less characteristic (Figs. 200, 201). The appearance of the vascularization is useful to differentiate it from other intracavitary tumors such as endometrial polyp and nodular endometrial carcinoma. Submucosal leiomyoma may also not infrequently show multiple development and coexist with other tumors such as endometrial polyp or endometrial carcinoma (Figs. 202, 203; also see Fig. 135). Recently, most submucosal myomas tend to be removed by means of operative hysteroscopy (Fig. 204) or resectoscopy under visual control (see Fig. 204a,b).

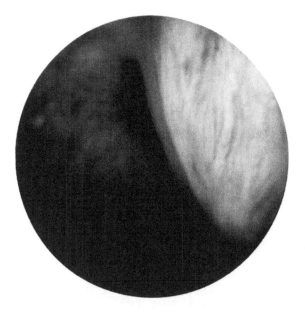

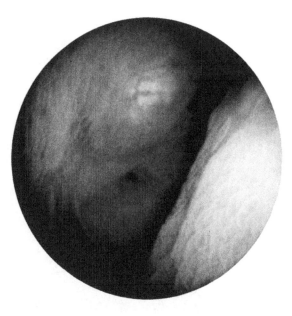

Fig. 189. Submucosal leiomyoma. Age 41. C.C.: Prolonged menstruation. The uterine cavity is distorted by a fairly large hemispheric nodule. The overlying endometrium resembles the surrounding tissue in the early proliferative phase in external appearance

Fig. 190. Submucosal leiomyoma. Age 42. Two submucosal leiomyomas are covered with translucent midsecretory endometrium with fine wrinkles

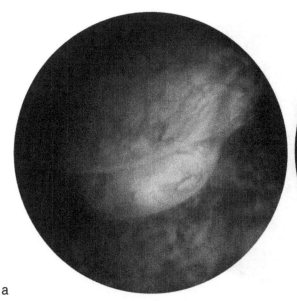

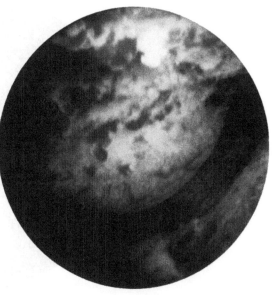

a

b

Fig. 191a,b. Submucosal leiomyoma. Age 39. C.C.: Prolonged menstruation. **a** The endometrium overlying a moundlike protrusion is atrophic, while thickened at the skirts. It is in the midsecretory phase. **b** Endometrial shedding during menstrual period is prominent at the skirts of a hemispheric nodule, while the endometrium overlying the nodule shows only sporadic blood spots

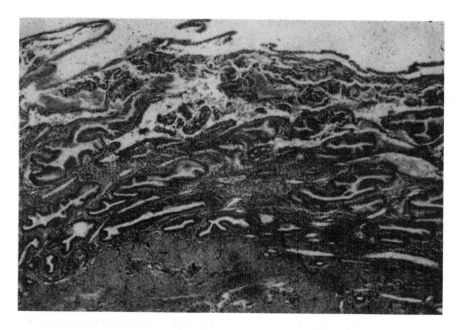

Fig. 192. Histology of the secretory endometrium overlying submucosal leiomyoma. The endometrium overlying a myoma nodule is fairly thick and provides a secretory feature. Glands are slanting because of oppression of the nodule

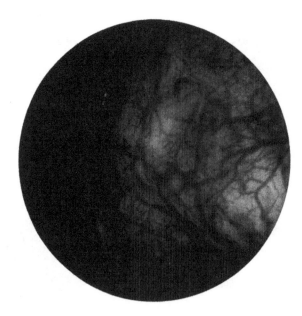

Fig. 193. Typical pedunculated submucosal leiomyoma. Age 50. The uterine cavity is full of a fairly large leiomyoma. The hairy vascular network displays in relief on the *whitish* ground of the atrophic endometrium against the *reddish* endometrium in apposition

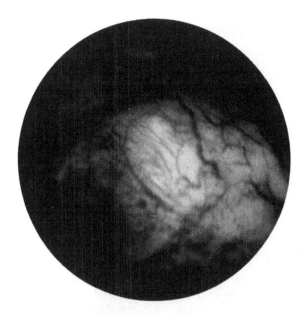

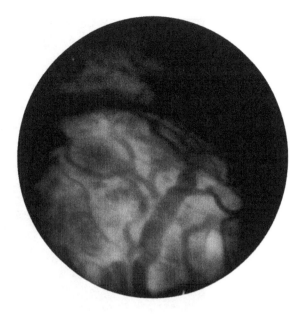

Fig. 194. Typical pedunculated submucosal leiomyoma. Age 47. The subepithelial vessels are a little thick but are regularly arranged

Fig. 195. Typical pedunculated submucosal leiomyoma. Age 29. Subepithelial vessels are dilated and closedly arranged. The endometria overlying and confronting the nodule are both thinned

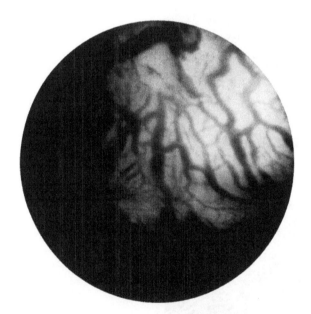

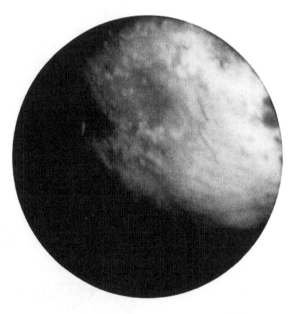

Fig. 196. Typical pedunculated submucosal leiomyoma. Age 50. Rather close but not atypical vessels display on the uneven surface of a nodule. It is necessary to discriminate this from nodular carcinoma of the endometrium (Figs. 121–125)

Fig. 197. Typical pedunculated submucosal leiomyoma. Age 60. C.C.: Postmenopausal spotting. The surface is *pinkish white* and scanty in vascularity. Bleeding originates from the surrounding endometrium, ulcerated by pressure, rather than from the myoma nodule

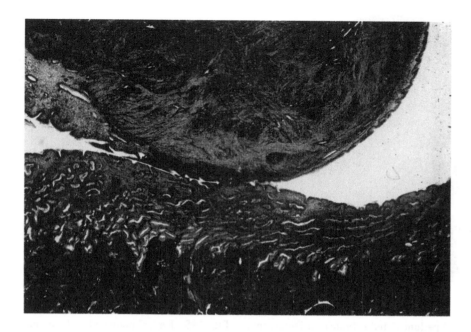

Fig. 198. Histology of the endometrium overlying a myoma nodule and confronting uterine wall. The endometrium overlying a nodule is atrophic at the top (*right*), while fairly thick at the bottom (*left*)

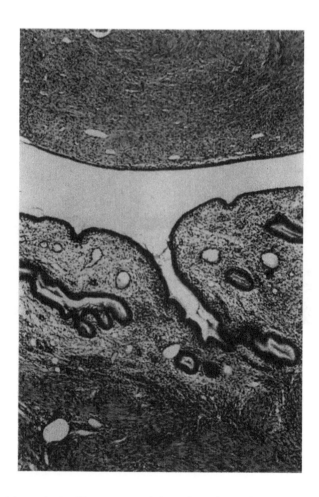

Fig. 199. Histology of a part in contact with myoma nodule and uterine wall. The endometrium investing a myoma nodule is very atrophic, while that overlying the uterine wall is rather thick

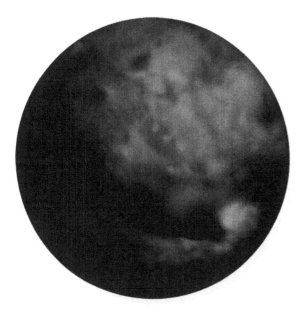

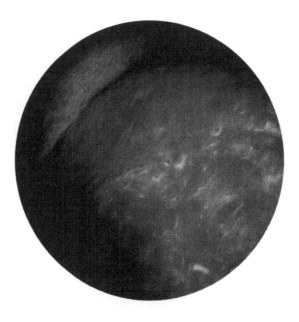

Fig. 200. Submucosal leiomyoma with profuse bleeding. Age 42. The surface is rough and ulcerated, showing blood spots in places

Fig. 201. Submucosal leiomyoma with engorgement. Age 46. The investing endometrium without shedding is *reddish* in color because of engorgement

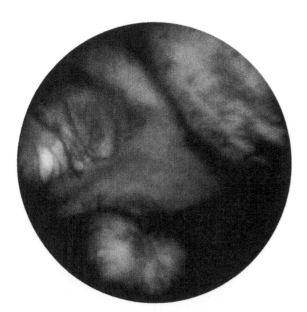

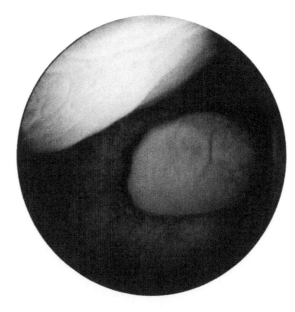

Fig. 202. Multiple submucosal leiomyomas. Age 47. Three myoma nodules with protrusions varying in extent can be seen

Fig. 203. Hemispheric submucosal leiomyoma (*upper left*) coexistent with a typical endometrial polyp (*right*)

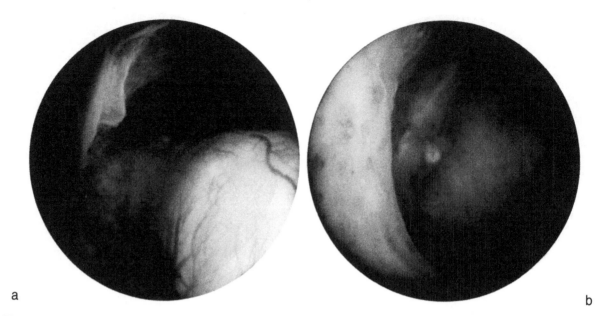

a

b

Fig. 204a,b. Submucosal leiomyoma with thick pedicle. Age 43. **a** This tumor could be removed by cutting off the pedicle. **b** On day 14 after myomectomy. The trace of the cut-off pedicle remains

7.2.8 Uterine Adenomyosis

Adenomyosis has been ordinarily estimated by imaging techniques that present abnormal thickening of the uterine wall without localized nodular formation. When the hysterogram shows irregular, serrated contours of the uterus, it becomes much more suspicious. However, it is the only time when the lesions are in direct continuity with the endometrial lining. As occluded lesions in the myometrium ordinarily do not display distortion of the uterine contour on hysterogram, it is rather difficult to diagnose adenomyosis by hysteroscopy as well as hysterograghy. Hysteroscopy can only confirm adenomyosis when the lesions have an entrance opening to the uterine cavity or lie just beneath the endometrial lining. The number, size, and shape of the openings, which appear as dilated indentation, vary from place to place (Figs. 205–209). Sometimes thrombus or ecchymosis can be detected around the openings immediately after menstruation (Figs. 210–212). Enclosed foci of adenomyosis can be seen *grayish-blue* in color through the thin lining.

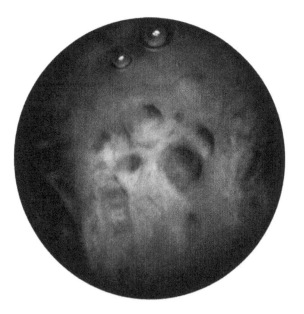

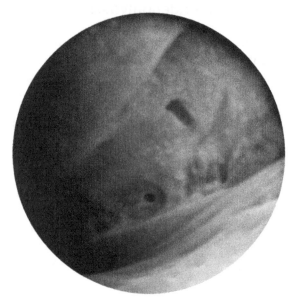

Fig. 205. Uterine adenomyosis. Age 47. C.C.: Dysmenorrhea. Round diverticula in various sizes can be seen at the fundus

Fig. 206. Uterine adenomyosis. Age 33.. C.C.: Dysmenorrhea. Deformed diverticula in various shapes can be seen at the fundus

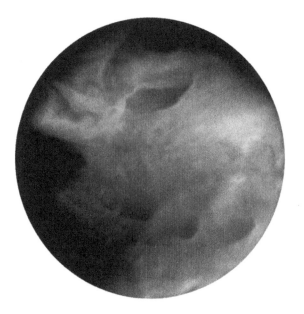

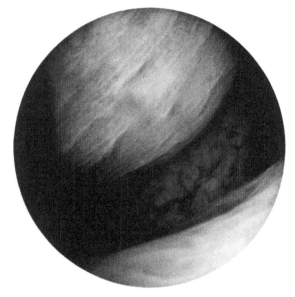

Fig. 207. Uterine adenomyosis. Age 48. C.C.: Dysmenorrhea. Diverticula in various sizes and shapes can be seen

Fig. 208. Uterine adenomyosis. Age 36. The uterine cavity is deformed by a slight eminence of the anterior uterine wall. On the surface of the eminence, several indentations can be seen on day 20 of the cycle

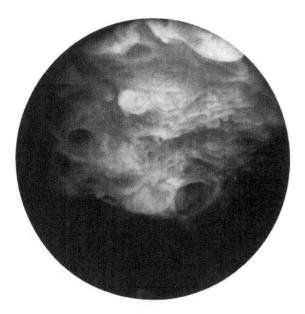

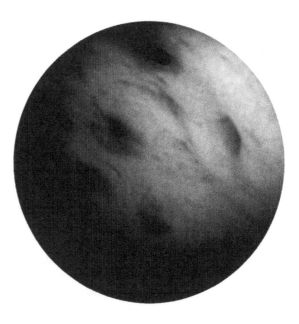

Fig. 209. Uterine adenomyosis under bleeding. Age 46. C.C.: Prolonged menstruation and dysmenorrhea. On day 9 after the onset of bleeding, the endometrium has been almost sloughed, leaving extremely dilated glandular openings

Fig. 210. Uterine adenomyosis under bleeding. Age 40. C.C.: Dysmenorrhea. Small blood clots obstruct the orifice of diverticula just after the stop of menstruation

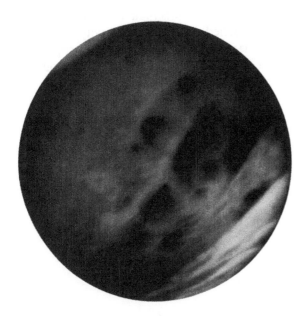

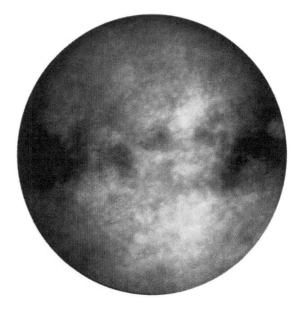

Fig. 211. Uterine adenomyosis. Age 43. C.C.: Prolonged menstruation. On day 7 of the cycle, the diverticula are packed with freckled blood clots

Fig. 212. Uterine adenomyosis. Age 23. C.C.: Dysmenorrhea. Although the lesions of adenomyosis come just under the uterine lining, they do not open onto the uterine cavity. *Grayish-blue* flecks and confined foci of adenomyosis can be seen through the endometrial lining

7.2.9 Endometritis

Because hysteroscopy invades the uterine cavity, acute endometritis is a contraindication owing to the dangers of spreading infection to the surrounding organs. Chronic inflammation is far more frequently encountered in the endometrium than acute endometritis. Abnormal uterine bleeding may be caused by chronic endometritis incidental to intrauterine foreign bodies such as IUDs and suture threads, neoplasmas in the uterine cavity, and inactive endometrial atrophy. Inflammation accompanied with foreign bodies and neoplasmas in the uterine cavity is described in each related section.

The postmenopausal uterus, absent from cyclic changes, is usually reduced in size. The inner surface is lined with thin endometrium and the cervix is narrowed. Thus, the senile endometrium provides a condition prone to infection. The hysteroscopic appearance of senile endometritis shows a more wrinkled or ragged surface with a sprinkling of blood spots than that of the normal atrophic endometrium (Figs. 213–218). Cystic glands sometimes can be concomitant (Figs. 219–221). Pathological lesions that necessitate a biopsy procedure may be nowhere to be found because the endometrium is too thin to obtain a sufficient specimen to evaluate its pathology.

Diagnosis of pyometra is easily made by an appearance of pus outflow from the cervical canal after uterine sounding or cervical dilatation. It is, however, most important to know whether the pyometra is primarily caused by cervical stenosis, complication of intrauterine malignancy, or merely idiopathy. The uterine cavity should be cleansed by enough lavage for clear vision in advance (Fig. 222a). The surface from which the pus coat is washed is coarse owing to shedding of necrotic tissue and looks *yellowish-red* in color (Fig. 222b). Hysteroscopy searches should be carried out all over the cavity to determine whether any other organic lesion is present. If first-look hysteroscopy has not been clear, it is recommended to perform second-look hysteroscopy after reduction of the inflammation by antibiotic medication (Fig. 222c–e).

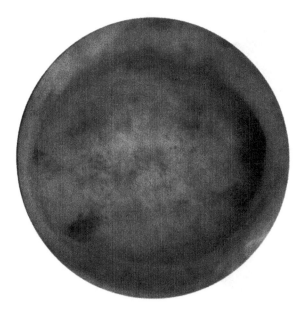

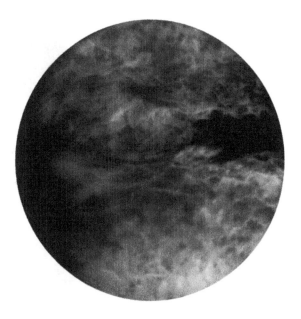

Fig. 213. Senile endometritis. Age 58. C.C.: Postmenopausal bleeding. The surface of the uterine cavity is flattened and *yellow-pink* in color, showing tiny blood spots

Fig. 214. Senile endometritis. Age 55. C.C.: Postmenopausal bleeding. The endometrial lining is rough, thin, and *yellowish-red* in color

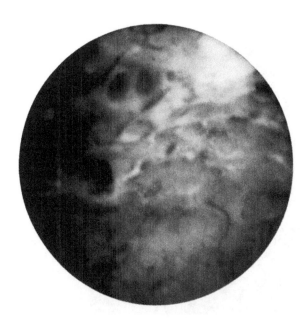

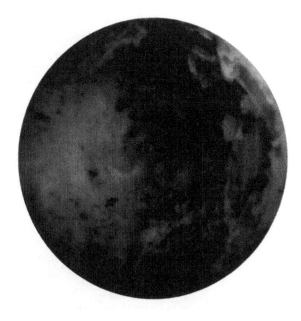

Fig. 215. Senile chronic endometritis. Age 79. C.C.: Continual bouillon-like discharge. The surface is rough, partly necrotic, and partly granular

Fig. 216. Senile chronic endometritis. Age 63. C.C.: Postmenopausal bleeding. The surface is rough, ulcerated, and studded by blood spots

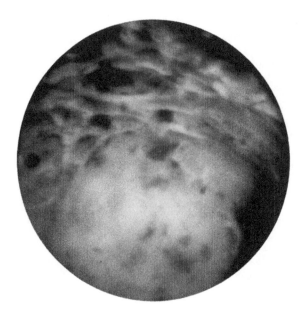

Fig. 217. Senile chronic endometritis with pyometra. Age 58. C.C.: Postmenopausal bleeding. The surface is covered with necrotic, ulcerated tissue, being spotted with blood

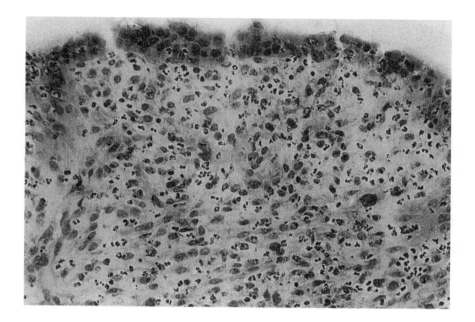

Fig. 218. Histology of nonspecific chronic endometritis. Age 70. If hysteroscopy diagnoses senile endometritis, curettage thereafter often cannot get a sufficient specimen to confirm the diagnosis histologically. This photograph shows a severe stromal infiltration of plasma cells and pus

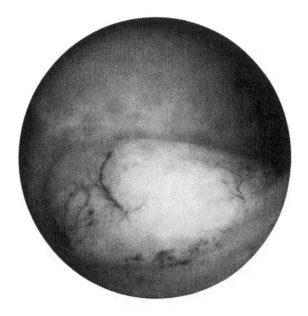

Fig. 219. Cystic gland of the uterine cavity in an older woman. Age 65. This patient has suffered from pyometra for 2 months. The cystic gland, protruding from the endometrial lining, is *white* and translucent

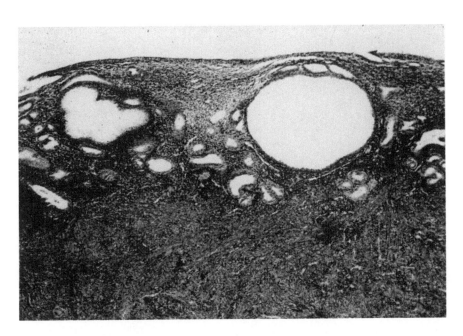

Fig. 220. Histology of cystic gland in senile atrophic endometrium. The cystic gland is thought to be a sort of retention cyst of the gland, the opening of which is obstructed by mild inflammation

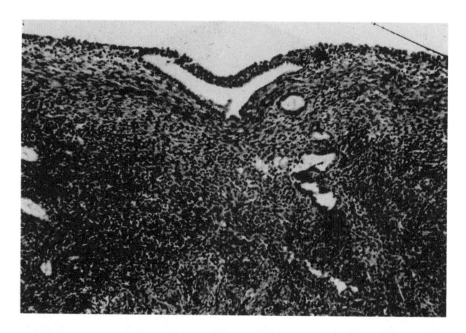

Fig. 221. Histology of mild chronic endometritis with cystic gland. The stroma is infiltrated by numerous pleomorphic cells. The subepithelial cystic gland is shrunk by formalin fixation

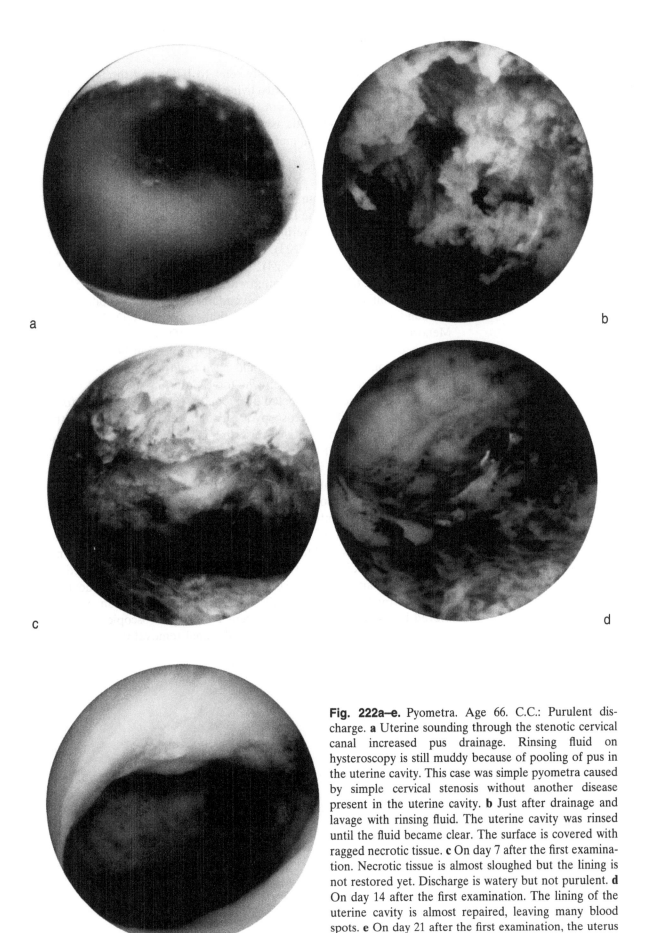

Fig. 222a–e. Pyometra. Age 66. C.C.: Purulent discharge. **a** Uterine sounding through the stenotic cervical canal increased pus drainage. Rinsing fluid on hysteroscopy is still muddy because of pooling of pus in the uterine cavity. This case was simple pyometra caused by simple cervical stenosis without another disease present in the uterine cavity. **b** Just after drainage and lavage with rinsing fluid. The uterine cavity was rinsed until the fluid became clear. The surface is covered with ragged necrotic tissue. **c** On day 7 after the first examination. Necrotic tissue is almost sloughed but the lining is not restored yet. Discharge is watery but not purulent. **d** On day 14 after the first examination. The lining of the uterine cavity is almost repaired, leaving many blood spots. **e** On day 21 after the first examination, the uterus has completely recovered its original order

7.2.10 Foreign Bodies

Intrauterine foreign bodies usually refer to IUDs and threads made from materials different from those of a living body, although in a broad sense they imply collapsed tissue organisms such as retained secundines, endometrial carcinoma, and endometritis as well. These foreign bodies occasionally may cause meno-metrorrhagia, increase of discharge, and infertility.

7.2.10.1 IUDs

There are usually few complaints associated with IUD use except an increase in the menstrual flow. The IUD properly fitted in the uterine cavity is gradually detached from the uterine lining with uterine distension by raising the rinsing fluid pressure (Fig. 223). Then, traces of the IUD appear as molds on the endometrial lining (Fig. 224). The surface of the IUD that has been in place for a long time may be dotted with calcium deposits (Fig. 225). Numerous tiny papillary projections of the endometrium with a capillary network surrounding the traces suggest focal irritation of the IUD (Figs. 226, 227). Menorrhagia and metrorrhagia in cases of IUD use may be occasionally provoked. These bleedings can be caused by infection besides preexisting organic lesions that otherwise would have been asymptomatic (Figs. 228, 229a,b). Postmenopausal women who forgot inserting their IUD a long time ago may be occasionally affected by pyometra (Figs. 230, 231). Before blind removal of the IUD, hysteroscopy is recommended to confirm whether abnormal bleeding is incidental to inserting an IUD or not. Postmenopausal bleeding or purulent discharge as well must be examined by using hysteroscopy to know if the cause of these uncommon conditions are independent of the probable insertion of an IUD.

Hysteroscopy is also a very useful method in the search for displaced, embedded, or fragmented "lost IUDs." Although a simple radiograph of the abdomen has helped to locate the presence of these "lost IUDs," the advent of hysteroscopy has facilitated location of partially embedded or fragmented IUDs as well as displaced IUDs (Figs. 232–236). For an embedded IUD, a simultaneous laparoscopy is recommended to know whether the device translocates through the uterine wall. Nonembedded devices can be safely retrieved by use of grasping-type forceps under hysteroscopic guidance. The translocated IUD may require transabdominal removal under laparoscopic control.

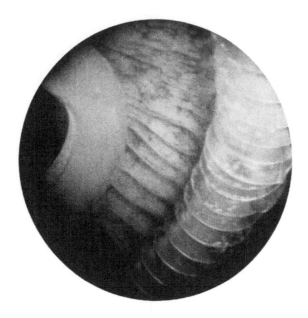

Fig. 223. Properly fitted IUD in the uterine cavity. Age 44. The endometrium is rutted by the wavy cast of Ohta IUD marks

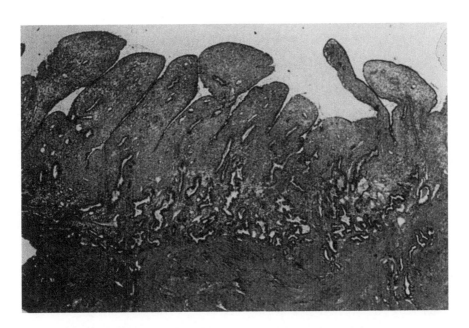

Fig. 224. Histology of the endometrium cast by Ohta IUD. This specimen has been fixed in formalin after removal of the IUD. The endometrial lining shows a wave resembling the cast of the Ohta IUD

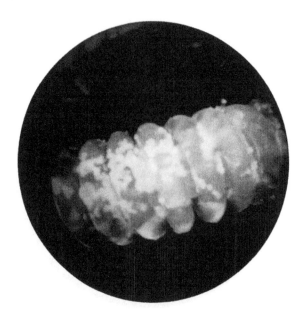

Fig. 225. Calcium deposit on the surface of IUD. Age 62. The IUD has been left in place for 28 years. The *white* calcium deposit occurs densely on the surface of the IUD

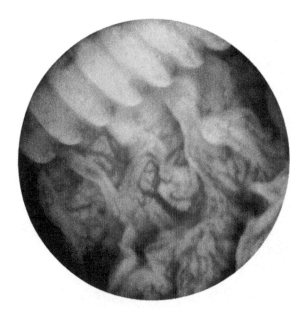

Fig. 226. Papillary projections of the endometrium stamped with IUD. Age 46. The top of each papillary projection, which provides a dilated vessel in the center, is swollen in a clublike appearance

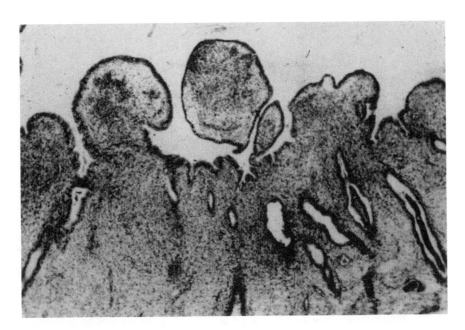

Fig. 227. Histology of the endometrium casted by Ohta IUD. The surface of the endometrium shows wavy swelling. Inflammatory changes in the stroma are not so conspicuous

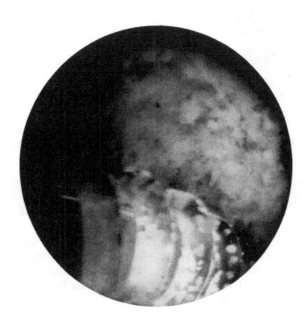

Fig. 228. Ohta IUD and chronic endometritis. Age 35. C.C.: Continual bloody discharge. This IUD was inserted 21 months ago. The IUD is dotted with calcium deposit. The surface of the endometrium oppressed by the IUD is rough and scattered with blood spots

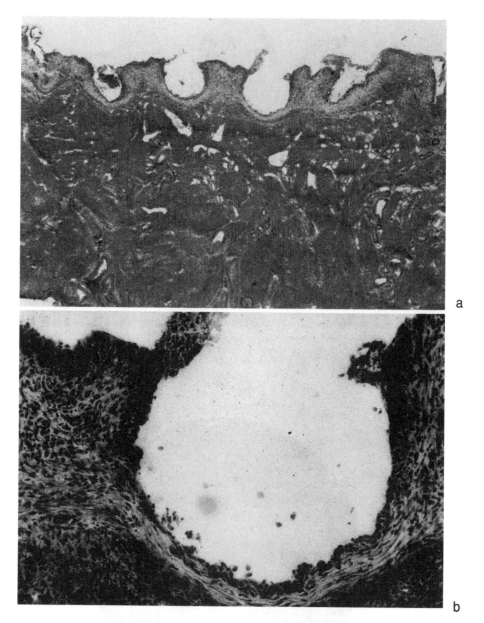

a

b

Fig. 229a,b. Histology of the endometrium molded with IUD. **a** This hysterectomy specimen, with IUD put on, was fixed in formalin. Fibrous projections grow between the lining epithelium oppressed by IUD and that free from oppression. **b** Highly magnified. Although the lining epithelium strongly oppressed by the IUD is atrophic, that free from the oppression proliferates with stratification. The structure at the border of both lining epithelia shows valvular flourishes

Fig. 230. Broken Ohta IUD and chronic endometritis. Age 60. C.C.: Postmenopausal spotting and purulent discharge. The patient had forgotten her IUD, which had been inserted 20-odd years ago. The IUD is fragmented. The endometrium is rough and partly necrotic

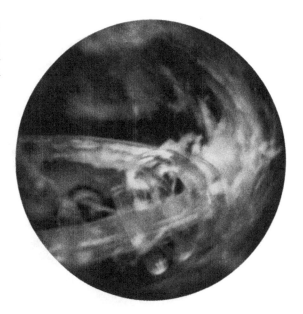

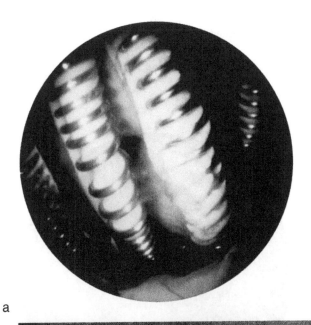

a

b

Fig. 231a,b. Five pieces of metallic IUD in the uterine cavity. Age 58. C.C.: Purulent discharge with lower abdominal pain. **a** Although it seems incredible, five IUDs were inserted at one time 22 years ago. It was not until pus had been cleansed by rinsing fluid that hysteroscopy found so many pieces of IUD as this in the uterine cavity. Five metallic IUDs were removed by grasping-type forceps under hysteroscopic control. **b** Five pieces of metallic IUD removed under hysteroscopic guidance

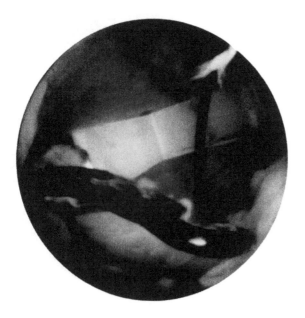 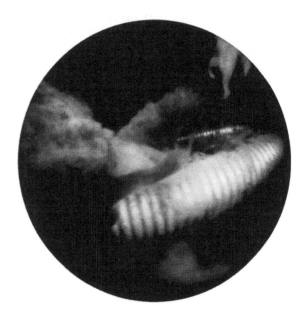

Fig. 232. Lost IUD. Age 44. The tail of a Lippes loop is retracted in the uterine cavity

Fig. 233. Lost IUD. Age 46. Part of a broken metallic IUD is embedded in the uterine wall

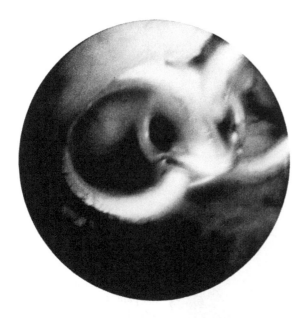 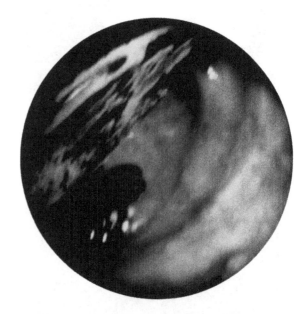

Fig. 234. Lost IUD. Age 42. Part of a fragmented 'Golden Wing' is embedded in the uterine wall

Fig. 235. Fragmented metallic IUD stuck into the cervical wall. Age 67. It was said that the IUD had been broken into fragments on blind removal using grasping forceps, leaving most of the fragments behind. One of the fragments sticks into the cervical wall

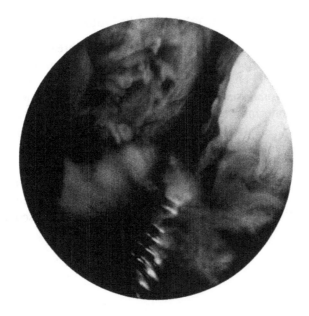

Fig. 236. Fragmented metallic ring stuck into the cervical wall. Age 23. On the occasion of blind removal, the IUD was broken into a few fragments, one of which is sticking into the cervical wall

7.2.10.2 Nonabsorbable Suture Threads

Although the use of nonabsorbable threads for conservative gynecological operation has been decreasing recently, particularly silk threads, which once had been used for suturing the uterine wall in cesarean section or myomectomy, can be rarely detected by using hysteroscopy in the case of abnormal uterine bleeding or infertility (Fig. 237). The silk threads that stick out of the anterior endometrial lining just above the internal os are in a tangle, being surrounded by granulation tissue with tints of *yellowish-pink* (Figs. 238–240a,b).

Other foreign bodies, namely the residue of HSG oily contrast medium, bone fragments, and laminaria stems, have been retrieved by grasping-type forceps from the uterine cavity under hysteroscopic control (Figs. 241–243).

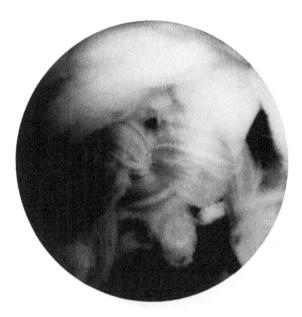 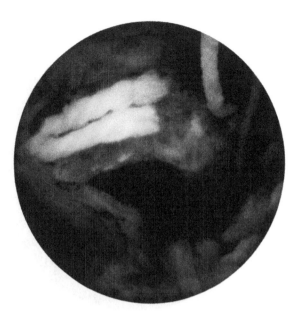

Fig. 237. Cat gut sticking out into the uterine cavity. Age 34. The patient underwent myomectomy in the fourteenth week of pregnancy, but suffered miscarriage after all, followed by continual bleeding. Knots of cat gut suture stick out of the broken uterine wall

Fig. 238. Silk thread in the uterine cavity. Age 22. C.C.: Continual spotting following cesarean section 7 months ago. Three pieces of twined silk thread surrounded by granulation tissue appear above the internal os

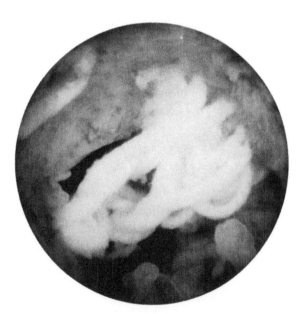

Fig. 239. Silk thread in the uterine cavity. Age 24. C.C.: Wish for childbearing. The patient underwent cesarean section 3 years ago. A few pieces of looplike silk thread dangle from the anterior uterine wall

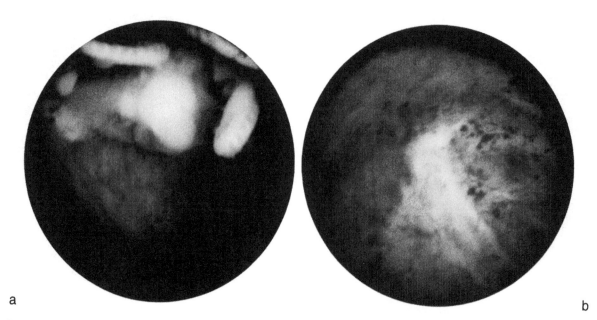

a

b

Fig. 240a,b. Silk thread in the uterine cavity with uteroabdominal fistula. Age 36. C.C.: Bleeding from abdominal fistula at the time of menstruation following cesarean section 18 months ago. **a** A few pieces of silk thread surrounded by granulation tissue hang from the anterior uterine wall. Hysteroscopy could not confirm the orifice of the fistula of the uterine wall. **b** The uteroabdominal fistula has completely closed since removal of the threads under hysteroscopic control, leaving a *whitish* scar

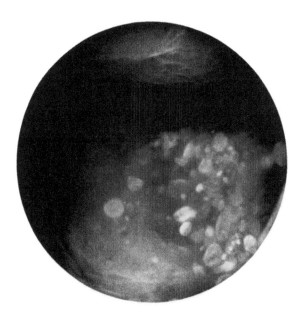

Fig. 241. Saponified oily contrast medium in the uterine cavity. Age 35. C.C.: Increasing watery discharge. The patient underwent hysterosalpingography 3 months ago. A cluster of twinkling *yellow* granules that are probably saponified oily contrast medium can be seen on the left side of the uteriine cavity

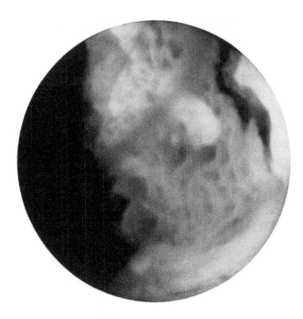

Fig. 242. Bony fragments in the uterine cavity. Age 31. C.C.: Metrorrhagia. This patient experienced an operation for legal abortion in the seventeenth week of pregnancy 4 months ago. Hysteroscopy shows a porous, hard, and ossified structure in the uterine cavity, although it is unclear whether the structure is retention of fetal bone itself

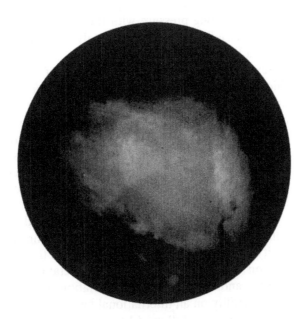

Fig. 243. Lost laminaria stem. Age 30. The patient underwent insertion of a *Laminaria* stem for legal abortion in the ninth week of pregnancy. A part of the stem was torn at the time of its removal, being left in the uterine cavity. The fragment of *Laminaria* was easily found by hysteroscopy and removed with grasping forceps

7.2.11 Traumatic Intrauterine Adhesions (Asherman's Syndrome)

Endocervical adhesions were described earlier. Most patients with traumatic intrauterine adhesions have a history of previous intrauterine mechanical manipulation in conjunction with pregnancy, such as missed abortion, incomplete abortion, molar abortion, legal abortion, postpartum placental retention, and cesarean section; also, they may also have a past history of conservative uterine operations such as myomectomy, metroplasty, and endometrial ablation. The main complaints are repeated abortion and infertility together with hypomenorrhea, amenorrhea, and dysmenorrhea. As the next step of examination, HSG is available for patients with these complaints. Hysterograms show irregular and rugged contours of filling defects located at the center or margin of the uterine shadow.

Hysteroscopy is very useful to evaluate and treat intrauterine adhesions. Hysteroscopy can reveal central adhesions that appear as a bridgelike column between the uterine walls (see Figs. 244, 245) corresponding with a central filling defect on the hysterogram and marginal adhesions which appear as crescent-shaped projections jutting out into the uterine cavity. Intrauterine adhesions are classified into three categories depending on the severity of adhesions. Mild adhesions are thin, filmy, and easily disrupted by the tip of the outer sleeve of the hysteroscope. The adhesions are composed only of endometrial tissue similar to the surrounding endometrium in color (Figs. 246–251). Moderate adhesions are slightly thick, lustrous and *whitish yellow* in color. The adhesions, composed of fibromuscular tissue, can be ruptured by rather strong pressure with the outer sleeve as well (Figs. 252a,b–254). When the adhesions are completely separated, two retracted stumps may bleed a little (Figs. 252b, 253b).

Severe (dense) adhesions, composed of connective or fibrous tissue, are thick, resistant, and look shiny and *whitish* in color (Figs. 255–257). The adhesions are single, multiple, or mixed with central and marginal ones in every case. In the case of severe multiple adhesions, it is difficult to bluntly divide the adhesions only by pushing the hysteroscope (Fig. 258). The only feasible technique is to gradually cut the fibrous tissue with scissors or laser beam through the operating hysteroscope under concomitant laparoscopic guidance. Still, it may be impossible to disrupt severe adhesions under hysteroscopic visual control.

The American Fertility Society has proposed a classification of intrauterine adhesions based on the hysteroscopic findings of the extent of the uterine cavity involved, the type of adhesions, and the menstrual pattern. This classification has been attempted in expectation of comparing the results of therapy and to evaluate the correlation between the treatment and subsequent fertility on an international basis.

Adhesiolysis is followed by insertion of an IUD in the uterine cavity to avoid readhesions for 2 months (Fig. 259). Concomitant hormone therapy to promote proper regrowth of the endometrium may be attempted. Most patients with mild or moderate adhesions restore their original uterine contour, increased menstrual flow, and fertility. However, one-third of the patients remain hypomenorrheic after synechiolysis and half of the patients who conceive experience abortion or premature delivery. In some patients with unsatisfactory prognosis after synechiolysis, hysteroscopy can reveal a focal endometrial atrophy or scarring with little cyclic function.

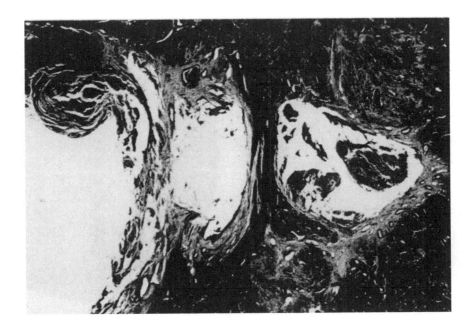

Fig. 244. Histology of intrauterine adhesions shown by Mallory trichrome stain. The left synechia, composed of an endometrial element, coexists with the right one of connective tissue

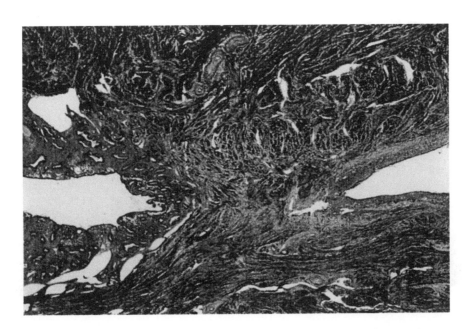

Fig. 245. Histology of myofibrous adhesion by phosphotungstic acid-hematoxylin (PTAH) stain. The adhesion is thick and tight because of fibromuscular connection

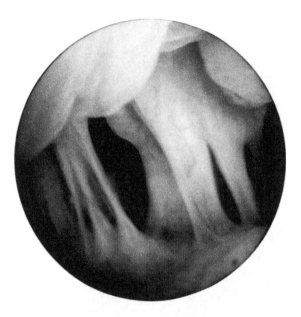

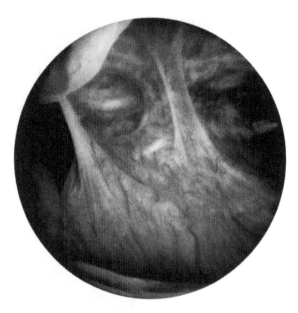

Fig. 246. Mild, multiple central adhesions. Age 43. C.C.: Hypomenorrhea after legal abortion. Several cordlike adhesions are soft, fragile, and can be broken even by increased pressure of the rinsing fluid

Fig. 247. Mild, multiple central adhesions. Age 39. C.C.: Hypomenorrhea after molar abortion. The adhesions are mild and extensive, but they can be easily broken by pushing with the tip of the outer sheath of the hysteroscope

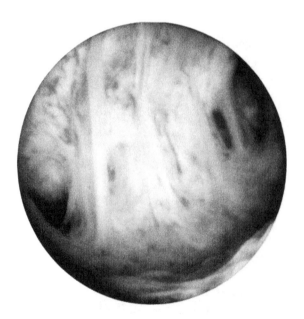

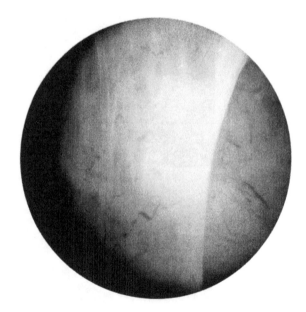

Fig. 248. Mild, multiple central adhesions. Age 22. These adhesions were found by hysteroscopy after intensive D&C of molar abortion. The broad adhesions are so soft as to be easily separated

Fig. 249. Mild marginal adhesions. Age 28. C.C.: Repeated abortion. A crescent-shaped adhesion can be seen on the right side of the uterine cavity. The structure is translucent and consistent with the secretory endometrium

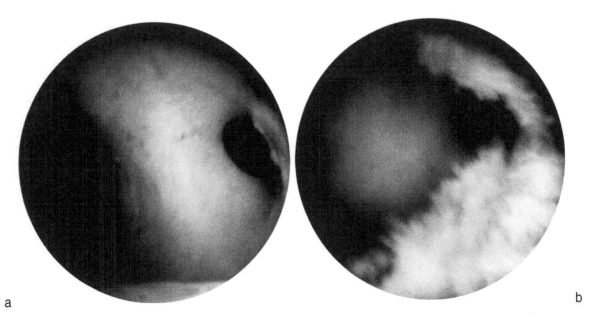

a

b

Fig. 250a,b. Column-shaped adhesion with broad base. Age 28. C.C.: Repeated abortion. **a** Her hysterogram showed a round filling defect in the midst. The adhesion is thick but soft. **b** After synechiolysis. The adhesions are easily lysed by pushing on the outer sheath, leaving fine ciliary stumps

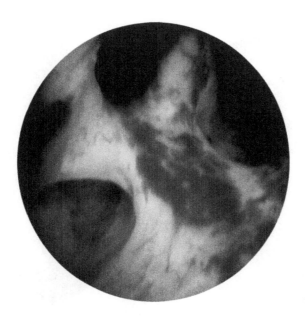

Fig. 251. Complicated mild adhesions. Age 37. The patient has undergone D&C many times because of adenomatous hyperplasia of the endometrium. The uterine wall is connected with three-pronged adhesions

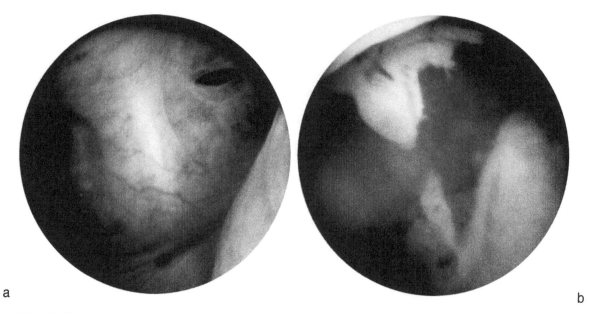

a   b

Fig. 252a,b. Broad moderate central adhesions. Age 36. C.C.: Infertility after legal abortion. **a** The left half of the uterine cavity is clogged with broad adhesions. *Whitish* luster at the midst suggests that it is of fibrous tissue. **b** Stumps just after blunt lysis. The stumps look rough but not fibrous, like the snapped end of a rod

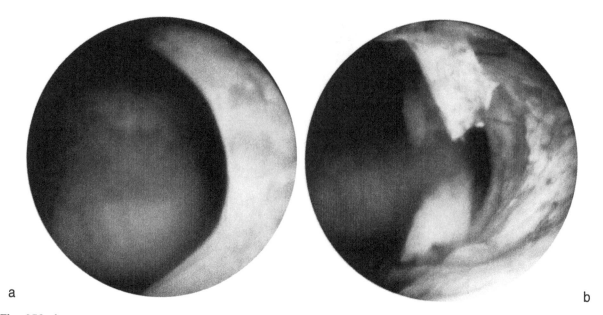

a   b

Fig. 253a,b. Moderate marginal adhesion. Age 34. C.C.: Repeated abortion. **a** Crescent-shaped adhesion begins to separate by oppression of the outer sheath. **b** Stumps just after blunt lysis. The adhesion is completely lysed, leaving retracted stumps on the uterine cavity

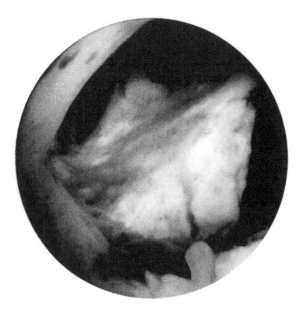

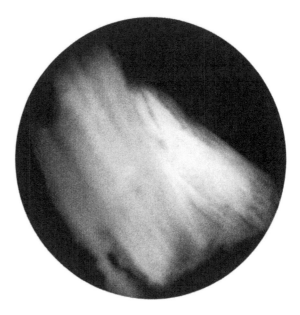

Fig. 254. Complicated moderate adhesions. Age 21. The patient underwent transabdominal myomectomy 1 month ago. Complicated moderate adhesions were separated under hysteroscopic guidance

Fig. 255. Coexistence of dense adhesion with a mild adhesion. Age 40. After evacuation of hydatidiform mole, columnar adhesions, which consist of a soft endometrial element and strong connective tissue, developed between the anterior and posterior uterine wall

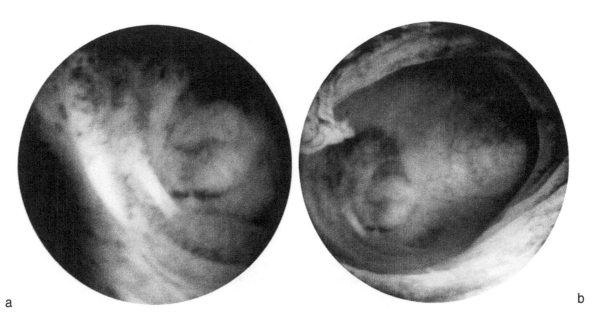

a   b

Fig. 256a,b. Dense marginal adhesions. Age 34. C.C.: Repeated abortion. **a** Connective tissues surrounded by thin endometrium occupy the right side of the uterine wall. **b** After blunt split of dense marginal adhesions, the uterine cavity has almost recovered its original configuration

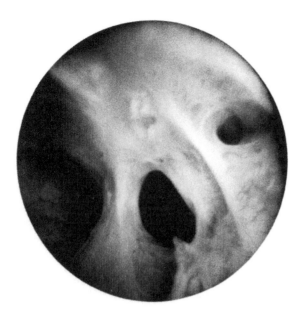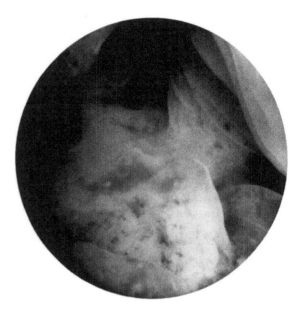

Fig. 257. Complicated dense adhesions. Age 28. This patient underwent D&C twice after molar abortion. Multiple adhesions can be seen over all the uterine cavity

Fig. 258. complicated dense adhesions. Age 45. Since undergoing D&C three times after molar abortion, the patient complained of hypomenorrhea. The uterine cavity is concealed everywhere by dense adhesions

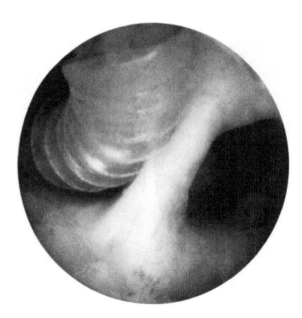

Fig. 259. Recurrence of adhesions after synechiolysis. Age 28. The patient underwent blunt adhesiolysis under hysteroscopic guidance and was inserted with an Ohta ring to prevent readhesion 2 months ago. New dense adhesion has developed near the IUD

7.2.12 Early Abnormal Pregnancy-Related Uterine Bleeding

Pregnancy of which preservation is expected has contraindicated hysteroscopy except for chorionic sampling. Although the diagnosis of pathological pregnancy, of which considerations should include missed or incomplete abortion, hydatidiform mole, and ectopic pregnancy, has been made by pregnancy test and ultrasonography, occasionally these results may be equivocal. Hysteroscopy is a feasible, harmless, and useful method by which we are able not only to detect the presence of products of conception but also to confirm their absolute absence in the uterine cavity lined with the decidua in the case of ectopic pregnancy. Besides, hysteroscopy enables us to differentiate these pathological pregnancies with abnormal bleeding from other diseases with hemorrhage such as dysfunctional bleeding and intrauterine neoplasm.

7.2.12.1 Retention of Secundines

In the case of retention of conceptual products with uterine bleeding, hysteroscopy can be easily carried out because the cervix is open and the uterine cavity distends without difficulty by using low-pressure rinsing fluid. In missed abortion, the gestational sac, which remains undisrupted but deflated, protrudes like a knoll into the uterine cavity, presenting a wavy surface (Fig. 260). It looks *grayish-blue* in color and is fragile. The endometrial lining (the decidua parietalis) is thinner than that of normal pregnancy and decreases in the properties of cribriform structure of the glandular opening (Fig. 261). Bleeding is mainly caused from the parietal decidua, which is partially peeled.

Hysteroscopic examination of the early phase of incomplete abortion indicates that fresh secundines are covered with blood clots in place of the vanished gestational sac (Figs. 262–265). After removal of clots using gently flowing rinsing fluid, the chorionic tissue with dendritic tentacles appears like seaweed with its outgrowth quivering in the liquid medium. The surrounding endometrium is mostly detached, which is similar in appearance to menstruation. Persistent uterine bleeding may occasionally occur in the case of unusually prolonged retention of conceptual products despite a negative pregnancy test and sonograms. In such cases, hysteroscopy is a simple procedure, enabling an immediate diagnosis and treatment under visual control. With the passage of time after abortion, the retained products of conception are localized, regressed, and organized, forming a prominence with a irregular or round surface (Fig. 266). They look *whitish-yellow* and are in an exquisite contrast to the thin surrounding endometrium with many blood spots.

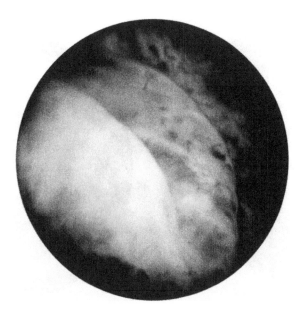

Fig. 260. Missed abortion. Age 25. C.C.: Slight bleeding after amenorrhea. The gestational sac, which is *grayish* in color and deflated, protrudes into the uterine cavity. Compare this with the intact, vivid gestational sac of normal pregnancy shown in Fig. 63

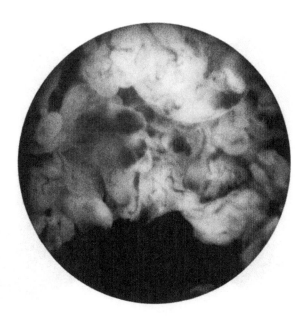

Fig. 261. The parietal decidua in missed abortion. Age 38. The decidua begins to slough, presenting a rough surface with blood spots

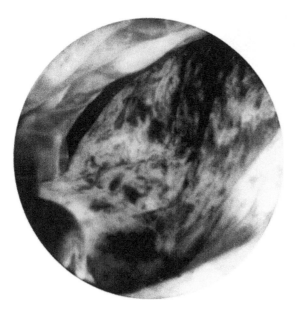

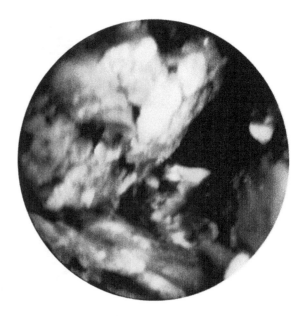

Fig. 262. Ongoing abortion. Age 37. C.C.: Profuse bleeding after amenorrhea. The structure mottled with *scarlet* and *white* is probably casting-off decidua

Fig. 263. Incomplete abortion. Age 40. C.C.: Profuse bleeding followed by continuous spotting. The irregularly shaped secundines are fragile and not vigorous

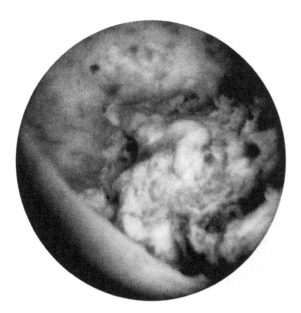

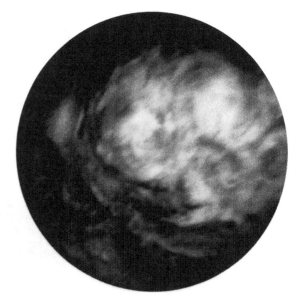

Fig. 264. Retained secundines. Age 32. Slight bleeding has continued for 9 weeks after induced abortion. A necrotic structure remains on the posterior wall. The surrounding endometrium is thin and sprinkled with small blood spots

Fig. 265. Retained secundines. Age 26. The patient has complained of menometrorrhagia since induced abortion 7 months previously. Although the round structure with the uneven surface is suggestive of non-epithelial neoplasm of the endometrium, histology of the curetted specimen showed retained secundines with indisputable shadow villi

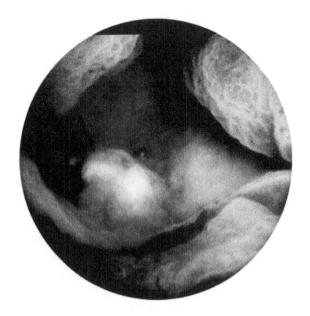

Fig. 266. Retained secundines. Age 31. C.C.: Prolonged menstruation after induced abortion. The patient underwent induced abortion 10 months previously. A small protrusion with *whitish-yellow* (*arrow*) hue showed organized secundines on histology of subsequent curet biopsy

7.2.12.2 Ectopic Pregnancy

Diagnosis of ectopic pregnancy with violent symptoms and typical signs is easy. However, when the disease has slight symptoms and goes through a sluggish process, the diagnosis consequently is difficult because of insufficient local signs. Diagnosis of ectopic pregnancy has been traditionally made by pelvic examination, D&C, culdocentesis, and ultrasonography. It becomes much clearer when hysteroscopy provides a useful view that the uterine cavity is empty despite a positive pregnancy test.

Tubal Pregnancy

Thanks to sophisticated vaginal sonography, now the presence of the gestational sac and fetus in the uterine cavity can be recognized in the sixth to seventh week of gestation. Therefore if there are no fetal elements in the uterine cavity despite a positive urinary human chorionic gonadotropin (hCG), ectopic pregnancy is very likely. When the fetal elements appear outside the uterus, the diagnosis is more precise. At hysteroscopy, the uterine cavity, which is easily dilated even by using low rinsing fluid pressure, is uniformly lined with the thickened decidua, and the gestational sac that should naturally appear in normal pregnancy in the eminence is absent. As far as progress of ectopic pregnancy is not interrupted, the decidua preserves an appearance similar to that of normal pregnancy (Fig. 267). As the pregnancy is discontinued, the decidua turns into an irregular pattern that shows irregular surfaces with partial blood spots (Figs. 268, 269). The uterine cavity in tubal pregnancy may occasionally be lined with the endometrium similar to that of adenomatous hyperplasia, which shows atypical vessels on the uneven surface (Fig. 270). At that time histology often shows the Arias-Stella pattern (Fig. 271). Uncommonly, when intermittent bleeding from the dilated tubal orifice can be seen, the diagnosis of the tubal pregnancy becomes more distinct (Fig. 272).

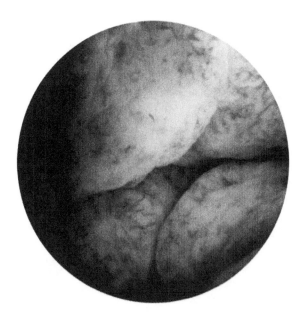

Fig. 267. The uterine cavity in tubal pregnancy. Age 32. C.C.: Spotting after amenorrhea. The uterine cavity, from which the gestational sac seems to be absent, is lined with the decidua-like endometrium, which is thickened and opaque with dilated glandular openings surrounded by fine vascular network on the surface. The left tubal pregnancy has continued without interruption

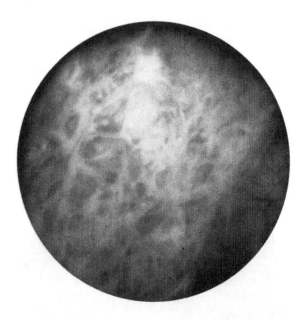

Fig. 268. The uterine cavity in tubal pregnancy. Age 38. When tubal pregnancy is prolonged without serious symptoms, characteristics of decidualized endometrium gradually decrease. Nine weeks have passed since the patient noticed bleeding after amenorrhea. The endometrium is thin, retaining the decidual feature with cribriform indentations of glandular openings. This case was right tubal hematoma without rupture

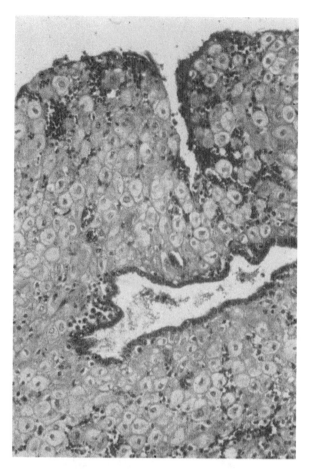

Fig. 269. Histology of the endometrium in tubal pregnancy followed by mild symptoms. The stroma is occupied by decidua cells interspersed by blood infiltration

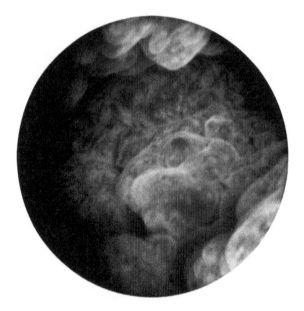

Fig. 270. The uterine cavity in left tubal pregnancy displaying an appearance closely resembling adenomatous hyperplasia of the endometrium. Age 32. The endometrial lining is rough, as in polypous hyperplasia. These appearances of the endometrium often show a Arias-Stella pattern on histology

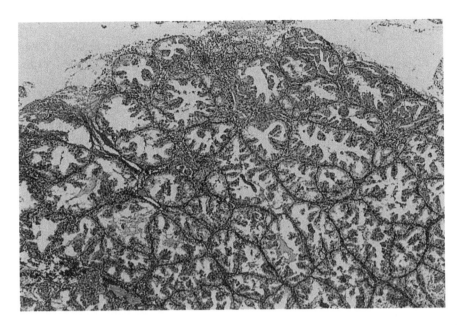

Fig. 271. Histology of the endometrium with Arias-Stella phenomenon. The glands are lined with papillary epithelial cells with vacuolated cytoplasm. The stroma is extremely oppressed back to back

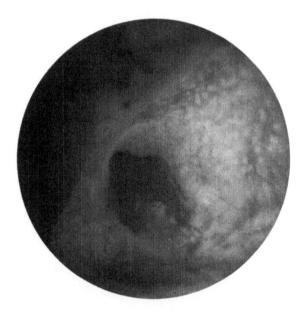

Fig. 272. Bleeding from the tubal orifice in right tubal abortion. Age 44. C.C.: Slight bleeding after amenorrhea. Hysteroscopy clearly perceives bleeding from the dilated right tubal orifice

Interstitial Tubal Pregnancy

Ultrasonography may be useful to diagnose interstitial pregnancy; the gestational sac before rupture can be seen just outside the uterine cornea in place of the uterine cavity. On hysteroscopy, the uterine cavity is empty, and also the irregularly dilated tubal orifice is filled with the complexes of products of conception mixed with blood clots (Fig. 273a–c).

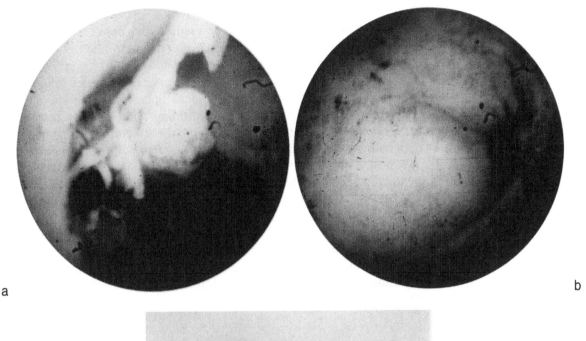

a

b

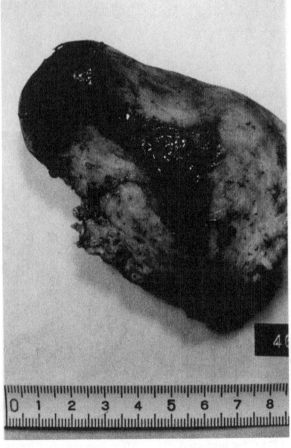

c

Fig. 273a–e. Interstitial tubal pregnancy. Age 36. C.C.: Continuous bleeding after amenorrhea. Because urinary hCG was positive and vaginal USG showed no gestational sac in the uterine cavity, ectopic pregnancy was suspected. **a** The dilated right tubal ostium is filled with a broken *whitish* structure. **b** The opposed left ostium is intact. **c** Hysterectomized specimen showed interstitial abortion without rupture

Cervical Pregnancy

Vaginal ultrasonography can also be useful to diagnose cervical pregnancy, although it is quite difficult to confirm it after its interruption as well as before that. Unfortunately we have no experience in hysteroscopic examination for uninterrupted cervical pregnancy. Usually cervical pregnancy cannot be recognized until conventional curettage, done under the diagnosis of ongoing abortion, induces much more copious bleeding. Although hysteroscopy must be carefully carried out so as not to injure the structure, the manipulation is quite easy because the cervix is open. The retained products of conception are located on a part of the wall of the cervix, showing an exquisite contrast to the surrounding folded endocervix; they appear as irregular processes with a *gray-brown* and uneven surface extending into the cervical canal (Fig. 274a). If possible, the hysteroscope is introduced into the uterine cavity without touching the lesion, and then it is proved that the uterine cavity in which conceptual products are absent is entirely lined with the decidua. One of the seven patients whom we had encountered was treated with local injection of MTX and then curetted, resulting in successful conservation of the uterus (Fig. 274b).

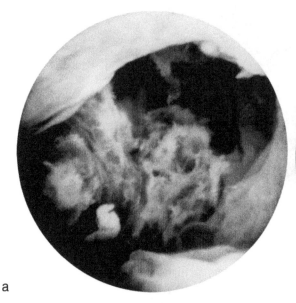

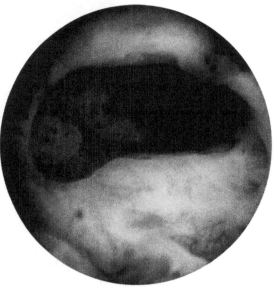

a

b

Fig. 274a,b. Cervical pregnancy. Age 33. C.C.: Copious bleeding during manipulation of D&C for suspected miscarriage. Copious bleeding suddenly occurred during the D&C. **a** Sophisticated hysteroscopy can easily find the tangled, necrotic structure in the dilated cervical canal. **b** After conservative treatment by regional injection of MTX, although somewhat dilated and flattened, the cervix is completely restored

Management of Trophoblastic Disease

Hydatidiform mole has been easily diagnosed by vaginal sonography. Hysteroscopy also gives us direct vision of translucent molar vesicles, which together resemble a bunch of grapes, *whitish-blue* in color (Fig. 275a,b). Second-look hysteroscopic examination a few days after molar evacuation is performed to verify whether all the tissue has been completely removed.

When destructive moles and choriocarcinomas develop after molar evacuation, they invade the myometrium, forming a hematoma. Although imaging techniques such as vaginal sonography and pelvic angiography may be available for the diagnosis, hysteroscopy also may be useful to view the lesions protruding into the uterine cavity; these present either a gentle eminence covered with the endometrial lining of *yellow-red* hues or blood clots mixed with necrotic tissue (Figs. 276, 277a,b). It is difficult to discriminate, by using hysteroscopy, between destructive hydatidiform moles and choriocarcinomas.

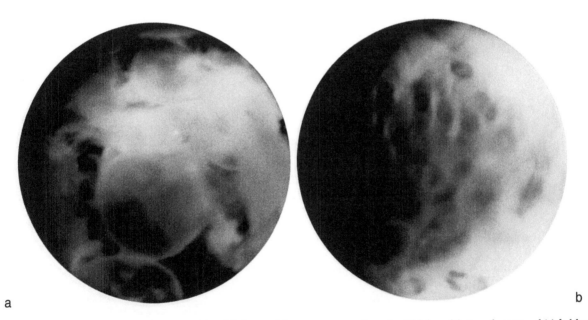

a   b

Fig. 275a,b. Hydatidiform mole. Age 25. **a** Molar vesicles appear as a bunch of blebs with translucent, *whitish-blue* hue. **b** Parietal decidua in a molar gestation. The decidua in a molar free part is thickened and edematous. Crowded, dilated glandular openings on the surface are prominent

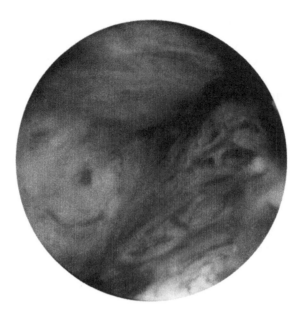

Fig. 276. Suspected destructive mole after molar evacuation. Age 30. C.C.: Bleeding lasting for 3 weeks after molar evacuation and persistent hCG in urine. Molar vesicles are absent in the uterine cavity, but hypervascularity of the left uterine wall presages trophoblastic disease invading into the uterine wall

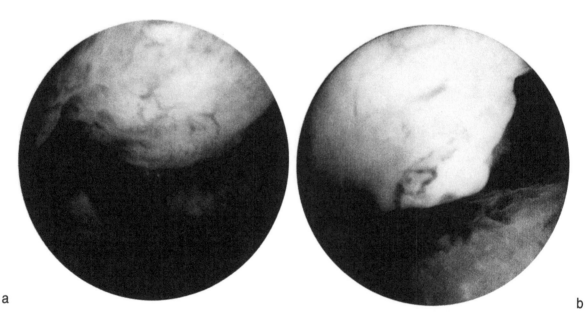

a

b

Fig. 277. Destructive mole after molar evacuation. Age 28. Hydatidiform mole was evacuated 3 weeks ago. **a** Round protrusion near the right uterine cornu suggests trophoblastic disease occulted in the uterine wall. Subsequent pelvic angiography proved the reliability of the hysteroscopic findings. **b** During systemic medication with MTX. Patient has undergone two courses of systemic medication with MTX. Rapid shrinkage of the tumor and decrease of urinary hCG after MTX medication demonstrated the usefulness of hysteroscopic diagnosis

Bibliography

Atlas of gynecologic endoscopy, 2nd edn (1995) Mosby-Wolfe, St. Louis

Baggish MS, Barbot J, Valle RF (eds) (1989) Diagnostic and operative hysteroscopy. A text and atlas. Year Book. Chicago

Barbot J (1989) Hysteroscopy for abnormal bleeding. In: Baggish MS, Barbot J, Valle RF (eds) Diagnostic and operative hysteroscopy. A text and atlas. Year Book, Chicago, pp 147–155

David C (1908) L'endoscopie utérine (hystéroscopie). These pour de doctorate en medicine (Jacques G, ed), University of Paris

Edstroem K, Fernstroem J (1970) The diagnostic possibilities of a modified hysteroscopy technique. Acta Obstet Gynecol Scand 49:327

Englund S, Ingelman-Sundberg A, Westin B (1957) Hysteroscopy in diagnosis and treatment of uterine bleeding. Gynecologia 147:217

Gaus CJ (1928) Hysteroskopie. Arch Gynaekol 133:18

Gribb JJ (1960) Hysteroscopy, an aid in gynecologic diagnosis. Obstet Gynecol 15:593

Hamou JE (1981) A new procedure and its original application in gynecology. J Reprod Med 26:375

Lawrence WD, Scully RE (1989) Pathology of the endometrium. In: Baggish MS, Barbot J, Valle RF (eds) Diagnostic and operative hysteroscopy. A text and atlas. Year Book, Chicago, pp 36–49

Lindemann HJ (1971) Eine neue Untersuchungsmethode fuer die Hysteroskopie. Endoscopy 3:194

Lindemann HJ (1980) Atlas der hysteroskopie. Fischer Verlag, Stuttgart

Mencaglia L, Perino A (1989) Hysteroscopy and microcolpohysteroscopy in gynecologic oncology. In: Baggish MS, Barbot J, Valle RF (eds) Diagnostic and operative hysteroscopy. A text and atlas. Year Book, Chicago, pp 114–120

Mikulicz-Radicki F, von, Freand A (1927) Das Tubenhysteroscope und seine diagnostische Verwendung bei Sterieität, Sterilizierung und Tuben evkrankungen Arch. Gynäkol. 123:68

Neis KJ, Brandner P, Hepp H (eds) (1994) Hysteroscopy. Thieme, Stuttgart New York

Neuwirth RS (1975) Hysteroscopy. Sanders, London

Nitze M (1879) Über eine neve Behandlungsmethode der Höhlen des menschlichen Körpers. Press. Wien, Wien Med Wschr. 24:851

Norment WB (1943) Study of uterine canal by direct observation and uterogram. Am J Surg 60:56

Norment WB (1949) Improved instrument for diagnosis of pelvic lesions by hysterogram and water hysteroscope. N C Med J 10:646

Norment WB (1951) A diagnosis test for tumors of the uterine canal. Am J Surg 82:240

Pantaleoni D (1869) On endoscopic examination of the cavity of the womb. Med Press Circ (Lond) 8:26

Peterson WF, Novak ER (1956) Endometrial polyps. Obstet Gynecol 8:40

Porto R (1974) Pneumocysteroscopy: instrumentation and technique. In: Sciarra JJ, Butler JC, Speidel JJ (eds) Hysteroscopic sterilization. International Medical, New York, pp 51–58

Rubin JC (1925) Uterine endoscopy, endometroscopy with the aid of uterine insufflation. Am J Obstet Gynecol 10:313

Schroeder C (1934) Ueber den Ausbau und die Leistungen der Hysteroskopie. Arch Gynaekol 156:407

Sciarra JJ, Butler JC, Speidel JJ (eds) (1974) Hysteroscopic sterilization. International Medical, New York

Seymour HF (1926) Endoscopy of the uterus: with a description of a hysteroscope. J Obstet Gynecol Br Emp 33:52

Siegler AM, Lindemann HJ (eds) (1984) Hysteroscopy: principles and practice. Lippincott, Philadelphia

Siegler AM, Valle RF, Lindemann HJ, Mencaglia L (eds) (1990) Therapeutic hysteroscopy. Indications and technique. Mosby, St. Louis

Speert H (1949) Endometrium in old age. Surg Gynecol Obstet 89:551

Sugimoto O (1978) Diagnostic and therapeutic hysteroscopy. Igaku-Shoin, Tokyo

Subject Index

Dextran 70 (Hyskon, Pharmacia) 3
5% dextrose 11
distension media 11
documentation chart 19

E
endocervical malignancy 38
endolymphatic stromatosis 111
endometrial ablation 24, 154
endometrial carcinoma 11, 18, 24, 87, 142
    cervical glandular involvement (stage IIA) 106
    cervical stromal invasion (stage IIB) 106
    diffuse — 87, 105
    metastatic — 105
    nodular — 87, 126
    papillomatous 87
    polypoid — 87, 88, 116
    polypous — 117
endometrial cytology 87
endometrial malignancy 23
endometriosis 74
endometritis 136, 142
    chronic — 23, 140, 145, 147
    nonspecific chronic — 138
    senile — 136–138
endometrium
    adenocarcinoma — 110
    adenomatous adenocarcinoma 87, 88, 90, 92, 95
    adenomatous hyperplasia 77, 85, 116, 166, 168
    adenomatous polyp 124, 125
    atypical hyperplasia 73, 77, 85, 86
    carcinosarcoma 110, 113, 114
    chondrosarcoma 110
    cribriform pattern 58
    cystic glandular hyperplasia 77, 116
    cystic hyperplasia 77, 83
    cystic polyp 118, 119
    early proliferative phase 50
    endometrial hyperplasia 77
    endometrioid carcinoma — 114
    focal hyperplasia — 85, 116
    high-risk hyperplasia 77
    involutional phase 56
    irregular shedding 64–66
    late proliferative — 67
    late secretory — 45, 56, 57, 71
    low-risk hyperplasia 77
    menstruating — 47, 49
    midproliferative 51–53
    midsecretory 55
    mixed mesodermal tumor 115
    nodular carcinoma 92–94, 99, 100, 107, 129
    nonepithelial neoplasia 110
    osteosarcoma 110
    papillary adenocarcinoma 100–102
    papillomatous carcinoma 74, 96–100, 103
    polypoid carcinoma — 107
    polypoid (focal) hyperplasia 77, 82, 89, 121
    postmenopausal 60
    regenerated — 48, 50, 51
    rhabdomyosarcoma 110
    senile atrophic — 61
    simple hyperplasia 77, 79
    stromal endometriosis 110, 111
    stromal sarcoma 110, 111
    tubular adenocarcinoma 87, 89, 95
    typical polyp 120, 121, 124
endoscope
    rigid — 4

F
fern leaflike fold 28
focal endometrial atrophy 154
fractional curettage 87

G
gestational sac 162, 163
Golden Wing 148
gonadotropin-releasing hormone (GnRH)
    analogue 73

H
Hopkins lens system 6
hormone replacement therapy 73
hydatidiform mole 159, 161, 173
hyperplasia *see* endometrium
hysterofiberscope 4, 8
    steerable — 9
hysteroscope
    flexible — 5
    Hamou's microcolpo— 8, 10
    liquid-type — 3
    needle — 8
    operating — 8, 154
    panoramic — 5, 15, 54, 96
    rigid — 5–7
    steerable — 8
    clinical indications — 23
    CO_2 — 11, 13, 14
    contraindications — 24
    diagnostic — 23
    first-look — 136
    flexible — 10
    liquid — 11
    operative — 4, 126
    rigid — 10
    second-look — 117, 136
    water — 13, 14, 44
hysteroscopy documentation 18

I

instant color print   20, 21
instrument
  flexible type   5
  rigid type   5
intrauterine foreign body   23, 136, 142
intrauterine neoplasm   161
intrauterine synechia   23
IUD   23, 142–144, 146, 154
  Lippes loop   148
  lost —   142, 148
  metallic —   147, 148
  Ohta —   143, 145, 147, 160
  translocated —   142

L

laminaria stem   150
  lost —   153
light-transmitting cable   6
local anesthesia   15

M

medroxyprogesterone acetate (MPA)   73, 86
menorrhagia   64
menstruating uterine cavity   46
menstruation   44
  anovulatory —   64, 67
  prolonged —   64
mesodermal malignancy   110
metallic ring   149
metroplasty   154
midcycle   53, 54
MTX   172, 174
myomectomy   23, 24, 150, 151, 154, 159

N

nabothian cyst   31, 60
nodular   91
non-epithelial neoplasm   164

O

oily contrast medium   150
outer sleeve   6, 7

P

paracervical block   15
pelvic
  active — infection   24
pill
  combined estrogen-progestogen —   73
  contraceptive —   71
plastic surgery of malformed uterus   24
plica palmatae   28, 33
polycystic ovary syndrome   89

polyp
  adenomatous —   116
  endocervical —   23, 32, 33
  endometrial —   11, 17, 23, 24, 98, 116, 126
  functional —   116, 117
  nonfunctional —   116
  placental —   116
  retrogressive —   116
  typical —   116, 122, 123
  typical endometrial —   131
polypectomy   23, 24
polypoid   89, 90
postpartum placental retention   154
pregnancy
  early —   58, 59
  ectopic —   161, 166
  interstitial tubal —   170, 171
  tubal —   23, 166–168
premenstrual spotting   71
pseudopregnancy   71, 73, 74
pyometra   24, 103, 136, 139, 141, 142

R

resectoscopy   126
rhabdomyosarcoma   115

S

saponified oily contrast medium   152
secretory phase   54
secundine
  retained —   23, 142, 162, 164
senile uterine cavity   61
squamocolumnar junction (SCJ)   38, 41
submucosal cervical leiomyoma   34
submucosal fibroid   13, 98
submucosal leiomyoma   11, 17, 24, 91, 126–129,
    131, 132
submucosal myoma   23, 116
synechiolysis   154, 157, 160
synechiotomy   24

T

tamoxifen   73, 76
thread   142
  silk —   150–152
  suture —   150
thrombi   64, 65, 69, 102
trophoblastic diseases   23

U

ultrasonography   166
uterine
  — adenomyosis   23, 133–135
uteroabdominal fistula   152

Lightning Source UK Ltd.
Milton Keynes UK
UKOW07f1837210316

270584UK00005B/33/P